Praise for Jonathan Kozol's *The Theft of Memory*
A *Library Journal* Best Book of 2015

"*The Theft of Memory* is a stirring, at times heartbreaking book about a brilliant doctor's valiant fight for his dignity following a devastating Alzheimer's diagnosis. Jonathan Kozol delivers this compelling narrative of his father's life and final years with extraordinary tenderness. Straight from the heart of one of our most thoughtful writers, this book is a revelation, offering both a celebration of the bond between a father and son and an insightful glimpse into the workings of our memories and the legacies we leave behind."

—Gay Talese, author of *A Writer's Life*

"For a number of reasons, many of us avoid thinking about old age, fading health, and death. Kozol's plainly and powerfully written book about his remarkable father is a notable and compassionate exception. It deserves to live on a small shelf with John Mortimer on Mortimer senior, Didion on Dunne, Bayley on Iris Murdoch, and Gawande on Gawande. . . . A fine and often eloquent book about holding on while letting go."

—Lawrence Hartmann, M.D.,
Past President, American Psychiatric Association

"Jonathan Kozol accomplishes something remarkable in *The Theft of Memory*: He preserves the essence of his father in the one place disease cannot touch him—on paper. . . . A soulful collage of a great man by his supremely gifted son."

—SUSANNAH CAHALAN, AUTHOR OF *BRAIN ON FIRE*

"The author's approach is shrewd yet warmly empathetic; he is curious about how the mind's gradual breakdown exposes its machinery, and raptly attuned to the emotional effects of these changes on his parents and himself. The result is a clear-eyed and deeply felt meditation on the aspects of family that age does not ravage."

—*PUBLISHERS WEEKLY* (STARRED)

"Readers familiar with the emotional toll exacted by a loved one with Alzheimer's will embrace Kozol's nostalgic, often heart-wrenching narrative as an important addition to the genre. A compassionate, cathartic, and searingly intimate chronicle of a crippling condition."

—*KIRKUS REVIEWS* (STARRED)

Also by Jonathan Kozol

The Theft of Memory

LOSING MY FATHER,
ONE DAY AT A TIME

Jonathan Kozol

B\D\W\Y
BROADWAY BOOKS
NEW YORK

Published in the United States by Broadway Books, an imprint of
the Crown Publishing Group, a division of Penguin Random House
LLC, New York.
www.crownpublishing.com

BROADWAY BOOKS and its logo, B \ D \ W \ Y, are trademarks of
Penguin Random House LLC.

Originally published in hardcover in the United States by Crown,
an imprint of the Crown Publishing Group, a division of Penguin
Random House LLC, New York, in 2015.

Library of Congress Cataloging-in-Publication Data
Kozol, Jonathan, author.
The theft of memory : losing my father one day at a time /
Jonathan Kozol.–First edition.
pages cm
ISBN 978-0-8041-4097-3 (hardback)–ISBN 978-0-8041-4099-7–
ISBN 978-0-8041-4098-0 (eISBN)
1. Kozol, Harry L., 1906–Mental health.   2. Alzheimer's disease–
Biography.   3. Neurologists–Biography.   4. Fathers and sons–
Biography.   I. Title.
RC523.2.K68 2015
616.8'310092–dc23
[B]   2014041699

ISBN 978-0-8041-4099-7
eBook ISBN 978-0-8041-4098-0

Printed in the United States of America

Cover design by Christopher Brand

10 9 8 7 6 5 4 3 2 1

First Paperback Edition

For Matthew

with deepest gratitude

CONTENTS

TO THE READER

This is a book about my father, who was born in 1906 and died seven years ago, in 2008. It is also a story about memory, and memory, among its many inconvenient and anarchic qualities, does not obey the rules of strict chronology. I have made no effort to disguise this.

My recollections of events in my father's life did not come back to me in single file like so many soldiers marching to a destination. They were prompted by the stories that he told me, those my mother told me, and those that I discovered in the documents and letters and memos to himself, and to other doctors, that he left behind, but most of which he never had a chance to organize before his memory began to fail. So a lifetime of experience has come to me in pieces that don't always fit together perfectly. I haven't tried to force them into sequence.

Other questions about memory—questions that my father raised, questions neuroscientists are posing now in more arresting ways—will be addressed at several points as they present themselves. Inevitably, uncertainties remain. I have had to learn to live with this.

The Theft of Memory

CHAPTER ONE

The Onset of an Illness

My father was diagnosed with Alzheimer's disease in 1994 when he was eighty-eight years old. He was a neurologist, with an extensive practice in psychiatry as well, and had taught for many years at one of Harvard's major teaching hospitals. It was one of the doctors he had trained who made the formal diagnosis of his illness.

The earliest signs of problems with his memory appeared about four years before. There would be times when he found it difficult to summon up the name of someone he knew well. Now and then, he'd also lose his purchase on a set of facts with which he wanted to support an argument. At other times, he'd briefly lose his sense of continuity in the course of what was otherwise a cogent conversation.

But my father had tremendous social competence. He'd navigate these awkward moments with congenial ease. He'd smile at his own mistake, then offer me perhaps a glass of brandy, and sit down and question me about my work, or tell me of a book that he was reading, or share with me an anecdote about his own career.

Sometimes he would light his pipe. (He liked to take his time packing the tobacco.) The aroma of the smoke as it rose up about him remains in my memory, comfortably intertwined with the sense of relaxation, confidence, and calm that I identified with all those other quiet and consoling conversations we had had over the years.

Then, in 1991, he started to get lost at night when he'd go out to take a walk in Copley Square, which is in the neighborhood of Boston where he and my mother lived. He'd come home three hours later and report perhaps that he had made friends with a couple visiting from London or Geneva, or that he had been at Buddenbrooks, a bookstore that was close to his apartment, and had had a conversation with a foreign student whom he might have met there. My mother would worry terribly, of course, when he was gone so long. His interesting narratives, I thought, were meant to reassure her.

In spite of his confusions, he continued to try very hard to get some work done every day. He had given up his medical practice by that time, but he was determined to complete some papers he'd begun—

summations of ideas that he'd developed in the course of his career on the neurological and psychiatric origins of certain forms of pathological behavior. A friend of mine, a teaching assistant at a local university, was helping him to organize his thoughts and bring coherence to his writing. On occasion, when my father asked, I would help him too.

It was not long after this, however, that my father's restlessness would overcome his capability for concentration. After an hour or two of work, he would push the pages aside, get up from his desk, put on his jacket and an overcoat, if it was cold weather, go down to the lobby of the building, and head off into the nearby streets for another of his evening journeys.

One night in 1992, he asked me to sit down with him in a room of his apartment that he'd been using to store an old examination table and some other items from his former office. He said there was something he needed to discuss with me. He told me that he hadn't yet decided whether it was wise to discuss this with my mother.

After he had closed the door, and both of us were seated, he started to lay out to me, in fairly graphic terms, what he described as "new and more specific indications" of problems he was having, which, he said, were "clearly neurological." He checked again to be sure the door was firmly closed and then began explaining to me what he meant by "more specific indications."

He said that he'd been having "spells"—he added that he did not mean by this the incidents of memory loss, which he called "amnestic spells," but something "of a different order altogether." He spoke of these as "brief attacks of interrupted consciousness" during which he recognized "a sudden cutoff from my own surroundings," "a definite blocking of 'capacity,'" lasting "maybe only for a millisecond or for several seconds or a trifle more." These episodes, he said, had been preceded in each instance by "an aura of impending danger" that he likened to the sense of warning epileptics often feel just prior to a seizure.

He did not say this with the urgent sense of self-concern one might expect a series of events like these would ordinarily arouse. Instead, he spoke as if he was attempting to position these events at a distance from himself, so that he could speak of them with the detachment of an interested observer.

"I can pinpoint this as a neurologist," he said, and he speculated that his recollection of what he'd been observing in himself might hold potential value for clinicians and researchers. For this reason, he plugged in his office tape machine, which he had used to dictate letters and reports on patients he was treating, and he recorded the remainder of our conversation.

He said that the amnestic spells were "clear-cut indications of degeneration of the cells in the cortex of the brain and in the hippocampus," and he showed me by the placement of his hand exactly where the hippocampus lies. He speculated also that "mini-strokes of very short duration," which he termed "a vascular phenomenon," were in all likelihood the reason for his episodes of interrupted consciousness.

Even more specific was the detail that he brought to the portrayal of that aura of anticipation that preceded this. He described it as "a feeling of uncommon and uncomfortable heat, 'a hood of heat,' as it were, that someone or some unknown force is drawing down over my forehead and my eyes..., as far down maybe as my chest or throat," and in another and, to me, more memorable phrase, "a feeling of impending desecration of my own autonomy—a premonition of my imminent removal from contextual reality...."

During that experience, or intermingled somehow with the loss of consciousness that followed, my father told me he was suddenly aware of "a very bright light," like that of "a locomotive bearing down upon you in a station." But then, after a moment of reflection, he corrected this from singular to plural—"No. Not a single light. Many lights"—and then, as if he was, step by step, retrieving the experience with more and more precision, he said, "I'm now recalling it more clearly. This was not a static light. It was more like flashing lights, coming up in rhythm. Thousands of lights shooting upward...and symmetrical. I remember that this frightened me. I needed you to know this."

It was the first time in the conversation that he let himself concede that he had been alarmed by this experience. "Those flashing lights are warnings of irregular electrical activity in the neurons, or between the neurons, which may terminate quite rapidly—or may not. In my case, it ended very quickly."

In the most recent incident, he recalled, "As I was coming out of this, I was aware of being very cold. There was cold sweat on my upper lip. Your mother was with me. She could see me shivering."

When I asked him where he was, he said, "In a restaurant. We were having dinner." As the attack subsided, he went on, "I heard a loud voice. 'Harry, are you hearing me?'" Although my mother realized that he wasn't well, he did not reveal to her what he'd just been through, because, he said, "Your mother's constant worrying is worse than anything my hippocampus may intend to do to me." I hoped my mother wasn't listening outside the door while he was speaking....

Having said this much, he seemed to be relieved, and he fell into a more reflective and more contemplative state of mind. Speaking now with less of the alarm he had displayed a moment earlier but once again in the more measured tone with which he had begun the conversation, he speculated that the light phenomena he had recalled (those "flashing lights coming up in rhythm...and symmetrical") "would have to have emerged from the occipital"—"from the posterior of the occipital," he specified, which he then explained to me, as if I were his student in a class on physiology, "is the region of the brain that processes our visual experience.

"This part," he said, "is something of a puzzlement. It's something that I've never seen in any of my patients...."

At that point, I suggested—not without some hesitation—that perhaps he ought to speak about these episodes with one of his colleagues. I asked him whether it was wise for him to try to fill the role of being his own doctor.

He looked at me for a long moment, searchingly, it seemed. Then he said that he intended to talk with a neurologist with whom he'd consulted on many of his cases—"I think I told you he was once my student"—but he took the opportunity to entertain himself by remarking that, although the man in question was "very bright" and "top-rate in the field," he was "a peculiar fellow, humorless and dour. Always was, as long as I have known him. I used to want to ask him what it's like to go through life without a personality."

He told me, in any case, not defensively or angrily but simply as a statement of determination, that he would see him at a time of his own choosing. "I want to ask you not to pressure me about this." He added that his confidence that I'd respect his judgment was precisely why he'd had this conversation with me, and not with my mother.

He waited another year and a half, but when he

knew the time was right he phoned his younger colleague and set up the consultation. There were no surprises. He knew what he would hear. The diagnosis by his former student was simply confirmation of what he already had discerned.

CHAPTER TWO

The Ends of Days

My father continued to live in the apartment for two years after that. It wasn't easy for my mother as his restlessness intensified and his memory progressively declined. The friend who had been helping him to organize his writings began to stay there overnight to relieve my mother's burden and to help my father deal with his confusions.

There were days when he would seem almost clear of mind. His conversational agility had not departed him. When he was in a tranquil mood, he could still be courtly with my mother. For all the tensions that simmered up between them, she didn't want to lose him.

Then, in 1996, he fell in the street in front of their apartment building on a rainy evening. A police car took him to the hospital. He had suffered a displacement of his hip. After surgery, when he came out of anesthesia, he had lost almost all recognition of what had happened to him, what his present life was like, or even where he lived.

After several weeks had passed, he regained a number of these memories, as well as a partial understanding of the situation he was in; but the time in which he'd been under anesthesia seemed to have left its permanent result in an unmistakable reduction of his cognitive capacity. He had to be placed in a rehabilitation center after surgery, and then, because of the suddenly accelerated diminution of his competence, I had to move him to a nursing home.

I was somewhat on my own in making these arrangements. Although I have an older sister, she had moved away from Boston more than forty years before and had settled in the Midwest with the man she married. She had two children (they were adults now) and an extended family of her husband's relatives, and many obligations and demands upon her time far from Massachusetts. For these reasons among others (my father had appointed me to be his legal guardian), decisions about choosing the right nursing home, working out the numbers for the costs this would entail, and making it a smooth transition fell to me, as did later choices that affected his well-being. My mother, of course, guided me as best she could in most of these decisions.

In the following month, my mother asked me

to come in and try to sort out some of Daddy's correspondence and his other papers. Several years before, he had sent me most of the case histories and related documents from his medical career for safe-keeping in my home, where they remained in large sealed boxes I had never opened. But there were other items he'd left here in his desk and in a metal filing case in a corner of the living room.

While looking through these documents, I found a picture of my father as a child. The photo was from 1912, when he was six years old. He was wearing knickers and a long-sleeved shirt, leaning against his father, who was wearing a formal-looking suit, a shirt with a round collar, and a broad and thickly knotted tie. My father's hand was holding his father's hand. The photo had a brownish tinge.

My mother was older than my father. He was ninety when he went into the nursing home; she was ninety-two. Although her body had grown frail, she was still a relatively healthy woman and still sharp and lucid in her thinking. But when my father had to go into the nursing home I saw a lost look in her eyes I'd never seen before. When I was sitting with her in her bedroom later in the week, she looked away from me, gazing out the window, across the river, at the Cambridge skyline, for the longest period of time. I had to speak in a loud voice to bring her back so she would see that I was there and speak to me directly. I showed her the picture of my father that I'd found. She said, "Your grandfather was a handsome man,

but no man that I ever met was as good-looking as
your father!"

My grandfather had come to the United States
ten years before that photograph was taken: the start
of a century that now was nearly at its end. He had
grown up in a village in the Ukraine, which was part
of Russia then. My grandmother followed him two
years later on a ship from Rotterdam to Boston.

Grandpa was a tailor but was earning very little
money at the time when she arrived, so she somehow
managed—I still do not know how—to rent or lease a
tiny store where she sold eggs and milk and ice and
soda, which was known as "tonic" in those days, and
some other groceries. I was close to my grandmother
when I was a child. She lived on Seaver Street in
Roxbury, which had been a mostly Jewish neighborhood until recent years. When I was at Harvard College, I would sometimes visit her on Friday nights.

My grandmother seemed to me a woman from
the Bible. She lit the candles in front of me and said
her prayers and gave me blessings and good dinners.
Even when I was twenty-one years old, she'd still put
candy Kisses in my pocket when I was about to leave.

When I became a teacher in the Boston Public
Schools in 1964, I would now and then bring students
with me to her house on afternoons or weekends.
My students were black children. My grandmother
had been hostile to black people when they moved
into her neighborhood. Their presence had frightened her at first. But the playfulness and sweetness

of the eight- and nine-year-olds I brought to visit her soon dispelled her biases and fears; they won her over with their innocence. She fed them and coddled them the same way she had done with me. They too got candy Kisses.

Now and then I brought my students to my parents' home as well, and, after my grandmother died, I did this more and more. My mother grew attached to certain children and would sometimes take the girls on shopping trips, then bring them home for tea. My father later helped some of my students go to college.

Many of my friends during the 1960s were political rebels and seemed to turn against their families for a time. Like them, I often had strong disagreements with my father, and I sometimes caused him needless worries and hurt him unintendingly; now and then, he could be harsh with me as well. But even in the last years of the 1960s and the first years of the 1970s, when my political beliefs became most heated and most radical and, I'm sure, more than a trifle grandiose, I found that I would turn to him when I was feeling insecure. He had a steadying hand.

As the years went by, however, and I found myself increasingly caught up in policy debates and in political forensics and was forced to travel a great deal, there were periods of time in which I didn't see my parents very much. Those were also years when I was writing books with a determined productivity that left me little time (or gave me an excuse to think that I had little time) to give them the attention they deserved.

Now, with my father in the nursing home and with my mother more and more confined to her apartment, with attendants to look after her, I felt angry at myself for all the opportunities I'd missed to be with them in the preceding years. As my father lost his wonderful proficiency with words, I wanted most to talk with him. As his memory failed and recollections of significant events that had taken place within the recent past appeared to have been lost for good, I wanted most to draw him out about the things he did remember.

My father had led a fascinating life that had involved dramatic changes in direction and, at one important moment, in the choice of his career. He spent much of his boyhood in South Boston, where his parents settled first after they arrived from Russia, and his later teenage years in Roxbury. He went to Boston English High, was admitted to Harvard in 1923, and earned enough to pay for his expenses by working at South Station as a soda jerk in his freshman year. He couldn't afford to live at college in a student dorm, so he was commuting from his home in Roxbury that year. Starting in his sophomore year, he lived at Stoughton Hall in Harvard Yard and tutored wealthy classmates who, he said, often didn't go to class and "drank more than they should" and, it seems, relied on him to get through their exams.

During his college years, he immersed himself in literature. He told me he had been especially attracted to Elizabethan poetry and theater; but he majored in psychology and spent much of his senior year working at a psychiatric institution called McLean and wrote his honors thesis—its title was "Religion and Insanity"—on the basis of his conversations with a schizophrenic patient he had helped to care for there.

In spite of his wish to continue with his interest in psychiatry, he went directly into Harvard Law School after college, pressured by his mother, who had wanted him to emulate his older brother, who had finished with his legal studies one year earlier. Only after traveling to Europe on a fellowship one summer to investigate the work of specialists in schizophrenia and meeting the man who coined the term, the great physician Eugen Bleuler, at his sanatorium in Switzerland, and later talking with the elderly neurologist Pierre Janet, an iconic figure in the study of hysteria, at the Hôpital Salpêtrière in Paris, did he make up his mind to give up law school and go back to Harvard College for two difficult semesters of chemistry, biology, and organic chemistry. By the end of that year, he entered Harvard Medical School, which was the start of yet another long and sometimes convoluted journey.

It had been hard for him to turn his back on expectations after he had been at law school for two years. To give that up because he had been stirred by his acquaintance with two elderly and eminent European doctors and was fascinated by the theories they discussed with him about psychopathology—and to do this at a time when he had yet to take the basic science courses that would be required for admission to the school of medicine—seemed very risky to his teachers and his mother. He did it anyway. Somehow the sheer bravado of this choice helped to fire up his energies and intellect enough so that he did it, not just with success but, as the years ahead would prove, with honor and distinction.

My father's life intensifies my feelings of respect for people who do not insist on too much certitude about the maps they're using and do not insist on knowing in advance what destination they'll arrive at in the ends of days. For many years he worked primarily in diagnosis of brain injuries and tumors, while he also grew involved with the brilliant Stanley Cobb, a pioneering figure in modern neuroscience, and the famously autocratic Derek Denny-Brown, a New Zealand-born neurologist, during trial periods of a medication called Dilantin, which proved to be a major breakthrough in prevention of the seizures undergone by epileptics. Later, he gravitated more and more into the practice of psychiatry. He was, according to his former colleagues, a sensitive clinician with unusual capacity to diagnose and to identify the separate elements of neurological and psychiatric illnesses in highly complicated and sophisticated people.

Some of these were well-known people—artists, writers, intellectuals, for instance. In Eugene O'Neill's last years, the playwright and his wife, a former actress named Carlotta Monterey, moved to Boston so that they could live close to my father's office. Beginning in the spring of 1951, they took a suite of rooms in a small hotel on Bay State Road diagonally across the street from the handsome town house where my father practiced. He saw O'Neill, who suffered from a neurological disorder, a tremor that had been misdiagnosed as Parkinson's disease, as well as from severe bouts of depression, at least once almost every day until O'Neill died of pneumonia in 1953.

He later entrusted to me many carefully packaged volumes of his daily observations of the playwright's state of mind and records of their conversations with each other, which reveal the growing sense of fondness that evolved between them. My father was, of course, much younger than O'Neill, and he looked even younger than he was. As unexpected as this may appear in the relationship between a patient and his doctor, and in particular in the case of someone as allegedly austere and undemonstrative in the display of his affections as O'Neill, it strikes me that he looked upon my father somewhat in the way a person might have looked upon a younger brother or a son. O'Neill had lost one of his sons to suicide about eight months before he had become my father's patient and had long been distanced from his other son and from his only daughter. Perhaps there was some kind of compensation in the close attachment he developed with my father.

I still have vivid recollections of the warm but often anguished references my father made to me about O'Neill, as well as his frustration with the playwright's wife, who, as I recall, competed with her husband for my father's time and loyalty.

I also remember the December day on which O'Neill was buried at a cemetery close to Boston. There were only three mourners at the grave site: the playwright's nurse, my father, and Carlotta. None of O'Neill's close colleagues from New York was present at the burial. My father later told me that they hadn't been invited by Carlotta, in keeping with her husband's wish that he be buried with simplicity and privacy.

After the playwright's death, my father underwent a period of grief that my mother felt was almost clinical in its duration and intensity. "I held his wrist within my hand as his pulse was failing and his heart stopped beating," as he recollected in one of the memos he was writing at the time. "I didn't want to let him go. I had a sense of desperation...." He later brought me and one of my college friends to see Long Day's Journey into Night when it began its run in Boston, but he grew distraught during the play and had to leave the theater to recover his composure.

His memories of O'Neill and other patients he

had treated were fading in and out, and growing less reliable, by the early 1990s; but his memory of what he did during the 1930s and the 1940s in the area of neurological impairment remained almost crystal-clear until the episode of injury and anesthesia that marked a sharp dividing line between the early phases of his illness and the onset of a deepening dementia.

Some of the most moving conversations that I had with him prior to his injury involved his effort to explain to me why memories of relatively recent happenings were beginning to be less and less accessible while others, such as memories of boys he knew and played with in first grade, and of the teachers he admired most at Harvard in the 1920s—Alfred North Whitehead, William McDougall, Abbott Lawrence Lowell, who was the president of Harvard at the time but also taught a government course my father took in sophomore year—were not only easy to recall but fresh and vivid, as if these were people he'd just seen or things he had just done.

"Lowell," he said, "had a little dog, maybe twelve or fifteen pounds. He'd walk with him in Harvard Square. At the curb, he'd hook his cane under the dog, lift him up, and carry him across the street...."

When he mentioned once that he'd studied with George Lyman Kittredge, whose annotated Shakespeare I relied upon when I wrote my thesis in my senior year, I naturally asked if he had had a chance to grow acquainted with him. "No," he said. "It was a large lecture class and, as I recall, I was just a soph-omore. Or, now that I think of it, I might have been a freshman. I would not have dared to try to talk with him. I can't imagine what I would have said."

But some years later, when he was in Geneva with my mother on the way to Zurich to meet Dr. Bleuler, he said he saw "the great professor" walk-ing by the lake. "He was just in front of us. I guess I must have stared at him, but I didn't have the nerve to introduce myself. 'Speak up, young man!' he said to me. I told him, 'When I was an undergraduate, you were my professor.' He was very kind to us and took us to have coffee. He even recommended a good place for us to eat. He said, 'The price won't kill you!' But when we looked into the window we could see that it was too expensive...."

My father took a lot of pleasure in recapturing these details, even while he recognized that he was losing track of many more important things that had happened recently. But it was the memories of his years of medical instruction and his retention of the terminology of neurological evaluation—because he used that terminology to describe his own condition—that I found to be particularly stirring.

Even after he had moved into the nursing home, he continued to retain some partial capability to speak about brain function. When he could not find a word he needed, he did not appear to be especially annoyed so much as curious and interested, like a sci-entist, to recognize in himself the same phenomenon he'd observed in others through the years. I could imagine him in the 1950s bringing young physicians with him on his rounds at Boston City Hospital or at the Massachusetts General, which was usually spoken of in Boston simply as the MGH, stopping at one bed, and then another, to discuss each case, and then arriving at a patient who presented the most perfect case of all to illustrate a point that he was making, even though the patient in this instance was himself.

Experiences like these had two effects on me. They heightened my respect for his capacity to reach beyond immediate predicament and find at least some elements of dignity and intellectual engagement in a situation in which others might have settled for self-pity. But they also were, of course, reminders of the probable prognosis for the future. The observations on brain function, as I knew, could not go on forever. Soon he would cease to be the doctor and remain only a case for other doctors to describe.

Once the injury to my father's hip was fully healed, he was able to stand and walk without assistance from the nurses and attendants. In nice weather I would take him out to walk along the road beside the nursing home. The road, which ran along a narrow stretch of water in a wooded and secluded area, ended at a tiny inlet in which ducks and ducklings floated back and forth and children would throw bits of bread onto the surface of the water just in front of them. In the other direction, we could walk along the woods and open fields for approximately half a mile to an elevation where there was an old stone chapel and a grove of apple trees.

These pleasant and unhurried walks brought back to me nostalgic memories of a time when I was nine or ten years old and my father used to take me with him on long evening walks around the neighborhood in which we lived, about ten miles west of Boston. The area, now thoroughly suburban, had been like a country village when I was in kindergarten. There was a cow named Daisy grazing on a hill across the street from us. By the time I was seven Daisy's meadow had been subdivided into lots for three brick houses. On several of the streets nearby, expensive-looking Tudor houses were constructed on the edges of tree-shaded properties that had been farms or large estates until the 1940s. Some of these houses were quite beautiful and stately and looked as if they had been built a hundred years before. On other streets, however, there were starkly modern mini-mansions, set on landscaped lawns with lighted terraces and pools, that looked too large and lavish for the lots on which they stood.

My father had a walking stick, with tiny copper medals nailed into its sides, that he had gotten years before when he went to Switzerland to talk with Dr. Bleuler. He liked to tap it on the pavement as we walked. Sometimes he'd stop and point it at a house we passed and tell me anecdotes about the owner.

He showed me once the mansion of a family that had been bootleggers in the 1920s—a member of the family had been "shot dead" by treasury agents on a beach near Marblehead, he said—but they had since achieved respectability as the owners of a liquor import company. My father didn't speak about these people in demeaning ways; he simply found the twists and turns within their lives intriguing.

More than a few of the people in the neighborhood had turned to my father for professional assistance during times of crisis in their own or in their children's lives, and he knew a great deal more than he was able to divulge about the sometimes unconventional arrangements and relationships within some of their families. Perhaps because I was a child, though, he shared a little more with me than he would allow himself to share with people of his age.

His observations on the private lives of certain of these families were presented to me, as I now remember this, in highly novelistic ways, as if these people were complex protagonists within a work of Thomas Mann, or Chekhov, or Flaubert. Disappointment, tragedy, and sometimes mild satire at a pretense of gentility in those who had amassed great wealth, but less refinement, in remarkably short periods of time, were commonly the richly woven strands of these narrations.

In later years my mother would explain to me some of the background of my father's state of mind at that point in his career. She said that he'd become increasingly ambivalent about the work that he was doing and the nature of the clientele he had attracted, which included many people who would travel here long distances from other cities to obtain his services.

A number of these cases tended to involve at least two members of a family whose behavior to each other might appear to be protective and affectionate but would, at the same time, be covertly toxic or sadistic. Simultaneously, within the tangled web of these familial pathologies, there might lie a neurological disorder such as a brain tumor. My father's diagnostic vigilance, as well as his gift for magisterial diplomacy in handling the tensions, for example, between children and their parents, or a husband and his wife, obviously served him well in these kinds of cases. Even so, according to my mother, he had grown uncomfortable about the role that he was asked to fill for many of these families, which seemed to him to be like that which in another age might have been filled by court physicians who had placed their expertise in subjugation to a very small and privileged elite.

This is not to say that he had ever turned his back upon his sense of obligation to provide his services to people of low income—or, indeed, to indigent people in the wards of Boston City Hospital, which served the poorest neighborhoods of Boston, as well as in the clinics of the Boston Psychopathic Hospital, which was affiliated with the MGH. But, to the degree that he allowed a handful of his patients to commandeer a disproportionate amount of his attention, and the degree to which he was obliged to draw upon his social skills in meeting their complex demands, I think he felt he was the victim of his own eclectic competence. And it was this, my mother said, that seemed to underlie those surges of impatience that would make him restless in the evenings and impel him to invite me to go out on walks with him.

My father's treatment of O'Neill did not begin until I was a little older. And his attachment to O'Neill, and the sense of honor that he felt at being asked to bring to bear the skills he had acquired in caring for the most respected playwright of his times, obviously compensated greatly for the feelings of frustration that he underwent in coping with Carlotta. Nonetheless, the sense of being in subservient attendance, which was engendered in my father by her overbearing ways, was a source of great discomfort to him.

I knew nothing of my father's discontent during those early years. I simply knew he liked me to go with him on his evening walks and that he talked with me more openly during those walks than he would do at other times. There was never any destination for our walks. I liked the aimlessness. We walked until his restlessness was gone.

Fifty years had passed since then. Now when we walked along the road beside the nursing home, he chatted with me off and on and usually made light-hearted observations about little things that captured his attention. He enjoyed the squawking of the ducks and ducklings and the sight of children who were feeding them. Sometimes I'd bring bread with me so he could feed them too. He liked to see how close they'd come before they grew afraid and circled off away from the embankment. But there were no more novelistic anecdotes. His ability to sustain a narrative of any length had now departed him.

Still, these were happy times for both of us. Now and then he'd take my arm and would point with his other hand at a wild rose or large sunflower or a graceful bird that floated over us. We'd walk until the reddish glimmer of the setting sun along the surface of the river was extinguished. He didn't tire easily.

CHAPTER THREE

A Fascination with Predicament

By his second year in the nursing home, my father's legs had grown much weaker and our walks became much shorter. Within the nursing home itself, he still insisted upon walking on his own, sometimes with attendants to assist him; but the sloping driveway outside of the building and the uneven paving of the hilly road below were difficult for him to walk without the risk of stumbling and injuring himself. Our evening walks along that country road would soon come to an end.

One night in the winter when I came into the living room where my father liked to spend his evenings, he was in a cheerful mood but thought that it was 1912. He spoke of "an enormous man" and then he made a reference to "the Gate of Heaven," an impressive-looking Roman Catholic church whose priest had been a good friend to his parents when they were, he told me once, almost the only Jewish family in South Boston.

The priest, as he had said, "used to come on Friday nights for dinner with my family. He loved my mother's cooking! He and Pa would have a glass of schnapps together in the kitchen before Ma put out our dinner on the table....

"One day, he took me with him when there was a big parade coming through South Boston. He put me on his shoulders so I could see above the crowd. There was this enormous man riding in an open car and waving to the people. I wanted to know who it was. The priest said, 'You are looking at the president of the United States. The man who's sitting in that car is William Howard Taft.'

"I realize now he must have been in Boston to campaign for reelection. I was six, so it had to be in 1912. That was the year when Theodore Roosevelt split the vote by running as an independent on the Bull Moose ticket. If my memory is right, that's the reason Woodrow Wilson was elected.

"Naturally, I didn't know this at the time. All I knew was that the priest had wanted me to share in the excitement. I was very fond of him. Some years ago I tried to look him up, but I was told that he had died...."

Now, in the nursing home, as his recollective

powers steadily declined, the detail that astonished him when he was six and its association with the kindly priest who took him on his shoulders were the parts that still remained to him.

On another evening later in the winter, my father didn't seem to recognize me when I first arrived, but then surprised me when one of the nurses came into the room. "I don't think I've introduced you to my son," he said. His voice had its old congenial sound, as if the two of us were at the Harvard Club for lunch ten years before and one of his physician friends had stopped by at our table.

Later that night, he talked about a boy named Danny Sullivan who was his playmate when he was in elementary school. At one point he asked, "Have you seen Ma?" He always spoke about my mother by her name or else he'd say "your mother," but he called his mother "Ma." I wondered at that moment if he thought I was his brother.

It wasn't sad to be with him, because he didn't seem to be unhappy. His confusions obviously troubled him but didn't seem to frighten him; and now and then there was a moment in which his responsiveness to an occurrence taking place around him in the nursing home—a medical emergency for instance—startled his attendants by its promptness and alacrity. One night, a woman who was visiting a patient suddenly collapsed and seemed to have gone into shock. My father got down on the floor and took her hand and pressed his fingers to her wrist to find her pulse. Appearing to be reassured, he stayed there at her side until one of the nurses had arrived.

Another night, as I was just about to leave, he took my arm and said something in Yiddish, which his mother spoke but which I hadn't heard him speak in many, many years. I asked him, "Daddy, can you say your name in Yiddish still?" He thought for a moment, then said, "Hershel Leben"—Harry Leo— and then put his arms around me and began to cry.

"It's been a good trip, hasn't it?" he asked.

"Yes, Daddy," I told my father. "It's been a beautiful trip. You made it good for all of us."

As often as possible, when I visited the nursing home, I'd try to bring my dog with me because her presence made my father utterly serene. She was a sweet dog, named Persnickety, a golden retriever whom my father used to play with when she was a puppy. She loved him dearly and, of course, placed no demands upon his cogency.

"Oh, there she is again," he'd say and reach his hand to stroke her head.

One night, when I let her off the leash as we were coming in the door, she raced around a group of patients in the hall, ran into the living room to the sofa where he liked to sit, and sat down in front of him.

She lifted her paw.

"Is Jonathan here?"

I was standing at the doorway still....

He'd usually say my name when I arrived. Or else he'd simply press my arm and hold me there in front of him and look hard in my eyes. "So how's it been?" he'd ask sometimes. If I told him I'd been in New York, he'd say something that was capaciously appropriate about the reason I was there. "Did you get it all done?" he might inquire. Or, on one occasion: "How are they treating you down there?" If I looked a little frazzled, or fatigued, he'd urge me to relax. "Ease it up," he'd say to me if he could see a worried look within my eyes.

When it was time for me to leave, he'd sometimes jab me gently in the arm. "Don't be a stranger now," he'd say, a phrase I'd often heard him use in decades past to say good-bye to someone he was close to—or, indeed, now that I think of it, to almost anyone who had been visiting our home.

One night he held my dog's head in his hands and studied her. A nurse who had a special liking for my dog said, "This one is an angel."

My father said, "Well, I'm not sure I'd go that far."

The nurse looked at my father with delight to hear him making this connection with her words. "What is she, Doctor, if she's not an angel?"

"*Practicing* to be an angel," said my father.

He continued holding her in front of him....

Only a week after that, he didn't seem to notice

31

when I came into the room. His eyes were shut. He looked as if he were asleep. But when my dog, who was standing right in front of him, grew impatient with his nonresponsiveness and began to lick one of his hands, he opened his eyes, stroked her head, and lifted up a cookie he'd been holding in his other hand, teasing her until she nearly climbed into his lap, her big front paws planted squarely on his knees, her soft brown eyes and dripping tongue directly in his face. His cheeks reddened, and in a boisterous act of self-defense he threw the cookie out across the carpet, watched her as she chased it underneath a chair, then reached for another cookie from a saucer on the table next to him and kept on playing with her in this way, exhilarated, as it seemed, by her enthusiasm for the game and by the little plaintive sounds she made when he held a cookie for too long.

"How old is she?"

"Almost seven," I replied.

He threw another cookie past the chair where I was sitting.

"There she goes!"

After he had given her the final cookie on the saucer, she came back from chasing it and settled down in front of him, curling up on the carpet at his feet and licking her paws carefully until she got bored with this and closed her eyes. Soon she was breathing heavily. My father closed his eyes as well. Before long, both of them were sleeping.

On another visit, when we stayed a little later than we usually did, she followed him when he was being taken to his bedroom. Once an attendant helped him to get into bed, Persnickety scrambled up and lay down on the linens next to him.

"Do you want to sleep with me?"

She made a grumbling sound.

"I think she may have been a lion once," he said to the attendant. "Would she let me comb her hair?"

She sat up suddenly.

"If you were smart," he told her, "you'd say yes."

She was looking down at him.

"Am I going to get a kiss?"

She licked him on his face.

"Where do you live?"

She licked him again.

"Being with this animal," he said to the attendant, "is conducive to religion."

Suddenly she sneezed.

Daddy said, "Gesundheit!"

For a number of years after coming to the nursing home, my father still could read aloud from printed words and, in the first two years at least, it generally seemed as if he understood them. I'd come in and find him sitting at a table turning the pages of the Boston Globe in a rather grand and authoritative way. By the end of the second year it became apparent that he no longer comprehended more than isolated pieces of a story, but the ritual of reading to another person seemed to be enjoyable to him.

He'd usually read stories from the paper or articles from publications like The British Journal of Neurology, which I would collect from his apartment when I visited my mother. He'd grow frustrated with himself if he turned two pages accidentally and would look back at the prior page again in order to assure the continuity. No matter how opaque the meaning might have been, he'd appear determined to complete a piece of writing when the text was there in front of him. Occasionally he'd make a statement of approval or of seemingly discerning disagreement.

One of the companions I had hired to give him more attention than the nursing home provided was a man named Alejandro Gomez, a Cuban doctor who had not yet passed the board exams in the United States and brought his textbooks with him when he spent time with my father. Since he was familiar with the language in the journals that my father read, he would try to offer substantive responses to comments that he made, even though he had to make what was, at best, an educated guess at what my father really meant to say. As imprecise and speculative as this reciprocity between the two of them might be, there was a feeling of engagement.

"I love your father," Alejandro said. He sometimes brought his daughter with him in the evenings.

She was a precocious ten-year-old, an inquisitive and outgoing child, and she liked to listen to my father, and she tried to figure out which way he might be going when he restlessly attempted to convey a clear idea. She was very good at doing this. When she was sitting next to him, he'd often lift his hand to touch her long brown hair.

Children of Alzheimer's patients frequently speak of the challenges they face in finding and retaining reliable companions who are not merely technically effective but also likable and interesting men and women who have a gift for making an emotional connection with the people whom they care for. I was fortunate in finding several people like that who knew how to stimulate my father's thinking process and who would respond to bits of memory he summoned up in ways that often stirred him to recapture other details.

Alejandro was perhaps the best at this. But there were others—a graduate student from Nepal who drove all the way from Amherst to be with my father two or three days a week in his first year in the nursing home, an artist from the seacoast town of Gloucester who wore a jaunty blue beret and had a spicy personality my father found enlivening, and a beautiful soul named Silvia Garcia, a fiery and strong-minded woman who became my father's closest friend and most determined advocate in his final years.

The staff at the nursing home, in contrast,

struck me, overall, as rather automatic, by-the-book, and sometimes quite impersonal in dealing with the patients. But there were exceptions. One of them was an extraordinary nurse, whom I will call Lucinda in order to protect her privacy because she told me many things in confidence that the nursing home officials probably would not have wanted relatives of people living there to know.

Lucinda was the first person with whom I spoke at any length on the day my father moved there. After a short period of time in which she observed my father's restlessness and his longing for companionship, she helped me to identify an agency that recruited healthcare personnel and was able to provide the kind of people she believed we needed to spend days and evenings with my father up until the hour, generally nine or ten o'clock, when he would go to bed. This was how we had found Silvia and Alejandro and the others I have mentioned. The agency, of course, added on a hefty fee for locating these individuals, so the cost of this turned out to be far more than I'd expected. Still, it proved to be a blessing for my father. With Lucinda there most evenings too, I knew he was surrounded by good people who were truly fond of him.

Right from the start, Lucinda went a great deal further than the call of her professional position. She quickly decided, for example, to go into Boston to get to know my mother, so that she would understand as much as she could about my father's life at home in the preceding years. She took an instant liking to my mother and she soon began going into town to spend an evening with her when she had no obligations at the nursing home. Sometimes she brought a chicken dinner she had cooked, so the two of them could have a meal together.

In the months in which my mother felt the most bereft at my father's absence, Lucinda helped to ease her sense of loss by sharing with her bits of news, and interesting things my father still remembered, which she thought my mother would appreciate. In this way, she came to be a source of strength to both of them.

The medical attention she lavished on my father was meticulous but always nicely humanized by the warmth of the relationship between them. One night, when my father's eyes had a little ooze in them and were slightly pinkish in the corners, Lucinda told me that he had conjunctivitis—very mild. She was applying small amounts of erythromycin ointment. While she was trying to do this, he pulled back his head and told her, "When I was a boy, sixteen, I called a taxi...."

"Where did it take you, Harry?" asked Lucinda.

"I'd like to ask you the same question!" said my father.

"But I'm not the one who called the taxi," she replied.

I liked the way she jumped right in and came back at Daddy with a good and lively answer of her own.

"I'd like...," he said to her, or perhaps to both of us, one evening when we were alone with him, then seemed to lose the direction of his thought and moved his lips but couldn't finish his idea.

"*What* would you like?" she asked him.

"I'd like to live for seven weeks," he said.

"Oh, Harry! That's not nearly long enough!" she said, looking directly at him with her glittery black eyes. "What would I do if I were here without you?"

On another evening, when Lucinda came into the living room after having been downstairs at a meeting with staff workers, my father looked right up at her and asked her if she had five dollars. Since she didn't have her purse with her, I took out a five-dollar bill and gave it to my father. Holding it in his hands and studying the wrinkled picture of the president in the center of the bill, he finally said, "This is what I paid to come here."

"Harry," she said, "I promise you five dollars wouldn't buy you more than a cup of coffee and a package of stale crackers in this expensive place!"

He tilted his head and gave her an appreciative look. A "twinkling smile" is the way I would describe that look of sudden gaiety.

My father's fondness for Lucinda was apparent in a letter that he gave her after he'd observed her at the far end of a corridor in a lengthy conversation with a youthful-looking man, who was probably a relative of one of the other patients there. "Dear Lucinda," he began. "It has taken me more time to write this than one might suppose. Advise: I hope your friend will profit from the opportunities we have all enjoyed. Please report to me on other gentlemen with whom you spend your time."

Lucinda took this in good nature and managed to pretend it was an indication of paternal thoughtfulness....

When I couldn't visit for a time because I was traveling or cooped up in my house working on a deadline for my publisher, Lucinda often phoned me or would dash off little notes to give me updates on my father's state of mind.

"Your dad went to sleep early tonight," she wrote to me one evening after she'd come home from work. "I'm told you brought Persnickety to visit him last week the night that I was off. Those visits mean so much to him! He'll talk about Persnickety for days after she's been here."

Now and again, Lucinda would surprise me by sending me a letter that my father wrote to me at her encouragement and, as I'm fairly sure, with some assistance from her, but in his own handwriting.

"Dear Jonathan," he began, in one of the first few letters that she sent me. "How have you been since our last visit, since our very last? Since I enjoyed it and I did, and do, the same. And I hope I will surely see you since our most recent. And I will gain some more impressions and good help and hope in these impressions and enjoy all your opportunities. Good for you and your parents and your friends and nearby visitors!"

In this letter, his handwriting had not changed very much from the time when he still lived at home. Although there were those obvious discontinuities, the meanings of his words were clear and each of the sentences was, in itself, coherent. Only in the final line did he seem to go off-track and forget the person he was writing to. Instead of signing "Love from Daddy," as he'd always ended letters to me in the past, he had signed the letter in the manner that he would have used in writing to a colleague: "Sincere Regards, Harry."

In another letter, written three months later, he began, "Dear Jonathan, please tell your mother she's too fine a woman to throw away her time on men she doesn't know." After asking me if I'd convey this message promptly, he continued, "I hope I shall see you soon, and both of us accordingly," but then concluded in the manner of a business letter as if, once again, he had forgotten, in the course of a few sentences, that he was writing to his son. "Your assistance in this matter would be much appreciated...."

Another time, when I had planned to visit (and Lucinda had, perhaps unwisely, told him to expect me), I was forced to change my plans because I had a cough and chest infection. When Lucinda phoned me the next afternoon to see how I was feeling, my father happened to be sitting in her office. He became concerned about me when he overheard part of her conversation. He wrote a letter which she sent me from her office fax machine as soon as she was done with work.

"Many of us are inquiring about someone who couldn't come to be with us. Herein: November the sixth. I hope you will feel better in the soon. Fate matters. We will keep in close dispatch." This time, he signed it, "Your one father, Daddy."

A slightly longer letter that Lucinda sent me, which wasn't dated but appears to come from the same period of time, conveyed the same clear recognition of the person he was writing to. It began, "To Jonathan my son," and then reported on some news that he'd received, or had imagined he'd received.

"No longer than an hour ago I received some information that might help improve my situation. But much has taken place beyond my capability to heal....

"Ma just phoned some moments ago. That did much to raise my spirits. It is too long since I've heard from her....

"Please provide whatever information on this matter you may have. Remember age and circumstance.

"I miss you."

Again, he signed it, "Daddy."

In spite of his confusion about who it was who

phoned him—if he had indeed received a phone call, it was probably from my mother—the letter was one of the most direct and self-aware that he had sent me up to now. There was no pattern or consistency in this. Sometimes it seemed as if the cloudiness that had descended on his understanding of the "here and now" of his existence opened suddenly, as in this letter ("much has taken place beyond my capability to heal"), and the cover-all expressions and discontinuities of meaning that I'd see in other letters disappeared almost entirely.

Six months later, Lucinda sent me yet another message from my father, this one, however, very different from the ones she'd sent before and not actually a letter but more like a memo, or a set of annotations, that a doctor might have made in observation of a patient.

"Repair repetitions," the memo began.

"Hope: Advise and continue treatment plan.

"Hope: in catastrophe.

"Legs: Recovery.

"Continue recent status of.

"Note: Loss of Certain Figures.

"List: History of HLK poses a number of several histories and multiple fine retardants...."

Even in the loss of continuity displayed in this and other memos he wrote later the same year, my father's attempt to identify his incapacities ("Repair repetitions," "Loss of Certain Figures") struck me as affirmation of the fact that he still was thinking in the terms of a clinician and organizing what he thought in the manner that had been familiar to him in his years as a practitioner.

Another memo that Lucinda showed me reinforced her sense, and mine, that he hadn't ceased to look at his condition from the vantage point of a physician, even while he also recognized that he was a patient. "In spite of various and said obstructions, I am trying to perform my duties and assist all local persons. There is little I can do except continue observations, viz., survey. How far is that other institution"—I believe that he was thinking of the MGH—"that attends to the same matters? I shall try again to ascertain today."

This was not the only time in which my father spoke as if he thought the nursing home might be a hospital or sanatorium in which he had some obligations ("duties") to perform. A few of his notations were, indeed, explicitly directive: "B.P. [blood pressure] straight across the board. Pt. [patient] now sitting very quietly. In no apparent pain. Release: uncertain. Please advise."

In another of his brief notations, my father made what seemed to be an indirect allusion to the sense of letdown and uneasiness that patients in a nursing home often undergo as the hours of the afternoon go by and daylight starts to fade. "I am under the impression," Daddy wrote in late December of that year, "that afternoons require of us greater sensitivity than presently provided. Reference made. Respectfully...."

My father was ninety-three years old on August 2, 1999. Although my mother had visited him as often as her strength allowed throughout the past three years, she wasn't feeling well enough to make the drive this time. Lucinda couldn't be there either, since she had to spend the evening at another nursing home that called her on occasion. So Silvia, who was spending more time with my father now than anyone except Lucinda, made plans with me to celebrate my father's birthday by ourselves. Naturally, I also brought Persnickety.

Silvia brought a chocolate cake with lemon icing that said "Happy Birthday Harry." In the garden behind my house the blackberries were ripe, so I picked enough to fill two small straw boxes and I brought them with me for our birthday party.

Persnickety, of course, became excited when the cake was taken from the box, so Silvia put the first slice on a paper plate and set it on the floor. After my father got the second slice, and then another—his appetite was very good, as usual—I showed him the blackberries I'd picked for him and he took one in his fingers, looked at it admiringly, and put it in his mouth.

"I love it," he said and reached out for another

one and then, in all, he ate perhaps about a dozen more.

The blackberries were at that perfect stage, plump and shiny, filled with juice, when they're most delicious. Persnickety, who loved to eat them from the bushes in our garden, suddenly became alert again. She sat up straight in front of him, gazing at him steadily and making that familiar sound of hers, a gradually increasing grumble, then a mild-sounding "whoof," which she knew that he would not ignore.

He chose one of the largest berries and he held it out for her. She made short work of it and looked at him for more. He teased her then, holding up another berry just above her nose, then lifting it a trifle more as her tongue got near, so that she had to climb on him before he would relent and pop the berry in her mouth.

As almost always was the case when Silvia or Alejandro was in charge of things, my father had been neatly shaved and dressed. Silvia usually dressed him in his chino slacks or corduroys and one of his nice jackets—beautiful but slightly worn tweed jackets, some of them with leather elbow pads, during the colder seasons, and a light blue seersucker jacket often on these summer days—and one of his deep blue shirts and handsome ties.

The juice from the berries had trickled on my father's lips. Silvia quickly found a napkin and wiped away the juice before it could run down across his chin and stain his shirt. Then he sat back in the sofa while Persnickety curled up on the carpet at his feet. The evening was warm. There were cricket sounds outside the window. My father looked about him with what seemed to be complete contentment.

Not every evening, naturally, was equally serene. There were times when undercurrents of concern—puzzling worries about my mother, for example—would intrude upon his sense of equanimity. Once, in the early autumn of that year, he suddenly looked up and asked me, "Is it true your mother's sleeping in a sewer?"

"No," I said. "She's sleeping in her bed."

"Where's she living?" he inquired.

"In the same old place—in the apartment," I replied.

"She's doing well?"

"She's doing fine."

"I'm glad to hear it," said my father.

A few nights later, he struggled for a long time to repeat a word I'd spoken, but could only summon up a word that sounded similar.

I asked him, "Does it madden you when you can't find the word you want?"

"That's it," he said.

"Something is playing tricks on you?"

"Exactly!" he replied.

He used one hand to draw a semicircle in the air. "It's like something...," then he broke off, but finally tried to finish the idea by saying "something in a circle?" I knew he hadn't made the point that he was after.

"Is that the word?"

"Not quite...."

"A globe? A sphere?"

He raised his hand, one finger pointed, as if I were almost there.

"A hemisphere?"

"That's it," he said. But then that moment of assertiveness was gone and whether I had really fixed on the right word at last—he'd often used that word, or "lobe," in speaking about functions of the brain—I wasn't sure at all.

Occasionally, from that time on, I noticed that my father found it difficult to speak about himself in the first-person pronoun. He knew the word he ought to use was singular. He knew it wasn't "you." He'd reach instead for "he."

"He's missed you," he might say to me when I arrived there after having been away too long.

Once, in answer to a question I had asked, he said, "He can't seem to recall...."

"'He' is 'I'?" I finally asked.

He looked as if he was delighted that I'd tried to stick a pin into the ambiguity of things.

"There's a connection...somewhere," he replied. Then, as if he'd had enough for now of the effort we were making to find sense in all of this, he made a joke out of his own bewilderment—"if somebody could only figure out what the hell it is!"

There was no apparent anguish in this flare-up of impatience. He simply shook his head a couple times, as people do to indicate that somebody they know who does peculiar things is "up to his old tricks." That clear blue gaze of unabated curiosity about his own condition still was there. Perplexity, the fascination with predicament itself, still drew him on—and drew me on as well. And once again, as when I was a boy of only nine or ten and he used to take me with him on those long walks in the autumn evenings, I felt that I was with my father on his journey still.

CHAPTER FOUR

"Can You Take Me Home with You?"

By April of 2000, my father had been living in the nursing home for three years and ten months. Even though he now could walk only for short distances without someone supporting him, Silvia and Alejandro and the others who took care of him knew it wasn't good for him to be sedentary for too long, which was unhappily the case with many of the patients who did not have private aides. He was sleeping longer hours now than he had done before and would often spend the morning in his bedroom but would spend his afternoons and evenings either in the living room or, in nice weather, outside on a patio.

There was a waist-high wooden fence surrounding the chairs and tables on the patio, which overlooked a sloping lawn where small brown rabbits hopped about and nibbled at the grass. The fence allowed me to unleash Persnickety so that she could wander freely from one group of people on the patio—visitors, staff members, or their patients—to another. But the rabbits proved to be a great temptation for her, and now and then, when someone didn't latch the gate that led into the patio, she would push it open with her nose and dash across the lawn in her big gallumping way in pursuit, always unsuccessful, of her small tormentors.

I didn't worry when she did this, because there was little traffic on the road below and she would quickly grow discouraged when she saw how easily the rabbits could outpace her. But my father grew uneasy if he noticed she had slipped away from us and if he then looked around and saw her running through the grass or sniffing at the flowers at the bottom of the hill.

Once, when we were sitting on the patio and she abruptly left his side and ran to the fence and used her paws to lift herself up high enough so that her nose was just above the upper rail, and looked down at a rabbit and made a plaintive sound, my father became agitated until I had gotten up and brought her back.

I told my father, "You had a worried look just now."

"Well," he said, reaching for her head, "he doesn't want any harm to come to her...."

His fondness for Persnickety posed a question for me later in the year when she developed a slight swelling on the upper surface of her nose. The swelling at first awakened no alarm—her veterinarian thought it was an inflammation, caused perhaps by allergens, and that it would subside. When it did not subside, but gradually hardened and increased in size, I brought her back to the veterinarian. The diagnosis this time was cancer in her nasal cavity.

By now, the swelling was so obvious that people working at the nursing home who had grown attached to her, and would often scrunch down on the floor (a few of the patients did this too) in order to pet and play with her, began to ask me what was wrong. And once Persnickety had undergone exploratory surgery, which required the shaving of a small patch of her fur and left an area of reddened skin exposed, as well as a line of stitches that extended almost to one of her eyes, it struck me as improbable that my father did not recognize these differences in her appearance when, as he always did, he held her head within his hands and studied her so closely.

The cancer was inoperable because of its location. A period of chemotherapy began in order to slow down the tumor's growth before it pressed against her optic nerve and started breaking down the architecture of the bone that protected her brain cavity. The doctor said that she was not in pain. But when the surface of her nose became inflamed, she would rub it with her paws and would sometimes cause the wounded area to bleed. Her doctor said she might have eight months, maybe twelve, possibly a little more, before she lost the satisfaction that she took in life.

One day, when the inflammation had returned and she lifted a paw to scratch the reddened area, my father quickly took the paw and held it in his hand so she couldn't raise it high enough to do her skin more harm. He didn't ask me what was wrong, but he looked at me, and then at her, with obvious concern.

I decided it was time to tell him what was wrong. I was confident he was going to outlive her, and I didn't want him to be disappointed suddenly when a friend who brought him so much happiness, and whom he almost always seemed to recognize the moment that she bounded in and took her place there at his feet, was all at once subtracted from his life.

But there was another reason why I told this to him now. I wanted him to keep on knowing me as long and as thoroughly as possible, and I knew this would not be the case if I presented to him only the most superficial aspects of my own existence ("happy talk") but steered away from everything that held importance for me. I wasn't married. I lived alone. Persnickety was my only real companion. I wanted my father to have the opportunity to understand, no matter how obscure and inchoate that understanding might turn out to be, why he'd now and then detect a look of sadness in my eyes that I didn't think I would be able to conceal.

Whatever he comprehended when I told him of the tumor, I had the feeling—and Lucinda said she was convinced of this as well—that there was something different in his manner now when he gently touched that area and traced the wound left by the line of stitches. If it was not comprehension of the danger she was facing, it was certainly solemnity. I think he knew that Persnickety, of whom he'd said so pleasantly two years before that she was "practicing to be an angel," was living with a shadow just above her forehead now. I know that line of stitches worried him.

One night toward the end of winter, as I was about to leave, my father asked me something he had never asked before.

"Can you take me with you?"

His capability to speak about himself in the first-person pronoun would resurface like that off and on, with no predictability. I avoided giving a real answer to the question. I think I came up with a vague equivocation. "It's a long drive, Daddy, at this hour...." Something of that nature. It bothered me that I couldn't find a way to answer him more honestly.

Before long, this developed into a familiar theme whenever he could see that I was getting up and putting on my coat to leave, even though I knew he had no recollection of the place I lived and I doubted whether he had any memory of his own apartment.

"Is it time for us to leave?" he'd ask. At other times: "Are we going home now?" When I'd say that I was going home but tried to find the gentlest way to tell him that I could not bring him with me, his eyes would sometimes cloud a bit or he'd simply look at me with wilted resignation. He'd follow me with his eyes when I went outside and passed the window near which he was sitting.

There was a television set on a maple table halfway across the living room. Once, when a patient turned it on, my father watched intently as a camera panned across the unmistakable façade of the MGH, the hospital in which he'd done his internship and, when he was older, had taken younger doctors with him on his rounds. He suddenly began to cry.

"Fight the fight!" he said to me.

I told him, "Daddy, you give me a lot of strength to keep on with my work."

"As long as I live!" he said and, reaching out one of his hands, he held me tightly by the arm.

Later that evening, when it seemed that he was growing sleepy, I took out my pocket watch to see what time it was. My father, apparently less sleepy than I thought, noticed the watch and took it from my hand and looked at it with what appeared to be consuming interest. His father had given him a beautiful gold pocket watch, which he in turn had given to me when I went to college. I kept that gold watch safely in my bureau drawer.

This one was an inexpensive and gold-plated version. He opened the cover and followed the second hand as it made its circle on the dial.

"Where are you living now?" he asked.

"Still in the same place," I replied, "right there up near Newburyport."

"Can you take me with you?"

"Not right now," I said.

"Why not now?"

I tried to give him a more candid answer than I'd given him before. "Daddy," I said, "my house is in an isolated area. It would not be good for you. I go away an awful lot. There would be nobody to care for you."

He studied the pocket watch a while longer and did not press me further about going home with me. Still, I knew that I had not assuaged his longing to come with me. Nothing I said was going to relieve that longing from now on.

Only a few nights after that, he looked up at me brightly when I came into the room and announced, "I'm Harry."

I replied, "I'm Jonathan."

"I know you are."

He stared very hard at me. Then he listed these four words: "Ma, Pa, brothers, sister...." (I should explain that, in addition to his older brother, who died before my father moved into the nursing home, he had a younger brother and a younger sister. His sister had died of leukemia when she was only forty-nine. His younger brother—I had decided not to tell him this—had passed away the year before.)

I didn't know what prompted him to say this. The words he had spoken seemed to come out of the blue. I wondered if he felt that, by announcing these few basic facts of which, if only at that moment, he was absolutely sure, he might be able to secure them in his memory.

On an impulse, I said my grandma's name to him in Yiddish: "Rivka."

He said it back to me in English: "Rebecca."

Another night, trying to draw out memories of things I knew he had enjoyed in years gone by, I mentioned one of the grand hotels in Northern Italy in the region of Lake Como, which he'd visited a number of times. He answered me immediately, but in Italian—"Lago di Como." Then he went on and spelled out each of those three words, then said the name again.

He would sometimes spell out other words he'd spoken—very short words usually. It reminded me of spelling bees in elementary school, in which a child got up from his chair, repeated a word dictated by the teacher, then spelled it out, then said the word a second time, then took his seat again. Is it possible my father was reverting to the days when he and his playmate Danny Sullivan were students in the first grade in South Boston? I knew that he'd been happy in his elementary school, although he'd told me long ago that he and Danny Sullivan had tried to burn the building down when they were in third grade.

"We set a fire outside the front door. I can't imagine why. Maybe we were angry at one of our teachers."

The fire did no damage to the building, but he said he got a spanking from his mother when she learned of what he'd done. He said she told him that, if he did not correct his ways, he was going to "grow up to be a hoodlum." (There were a lot of "hoodlums" in South Boston in those days, he said.) He told me the story several times. In spite of the spanking, he seemed to enjoy this memory tremendously.

Sadder times continued too. When I told my father once that I'd be away two weeks because I had to go to California and New York, he asked me, "Can you take me with you?"

"It would be awfully hard to do that, Daddy," I replied.

"Why?" he said. "Couldn't you try?"

"I'll be on airplanes," I explained. "It would be impossible."

"Can't you try?"

"No, Daddy. I can't do it."

It wasn't easy to be so direct with him at last but, when he pressed the point this time, I decided that I shouldn't string him out with tentative and vaguely worded answers anymore. As with the dilemma I had faced about Persnickety, I did not want to tell my father lies.

His adamant persistence on this matter, even though it made things difficult for me, was nonetheless a keen reminder that he had resisted that extreme passivity, that pattern of abject capitulation to decisions made by others, that is commonly induced in patients by the governance arrangements and the feelings of captivity that are familiar in a nursing home to which Alzheimer's patients and other patients stricken with dementia are confined. It seemed, indeed, that he was so determined to devise a way to get out of this institution that he did a lot of thinking to develop various ingenious plans for doing it.

One night, for example, when the two of us were sitting on the sofa and no one else was near, he leaned forward and proposed to me a way that we might pull it off. "When I need to, I'll come out"—he nodded toward the door that led out to the patio—"and I'll say, 'My son is coming for me.'" Then, as he had worked this out, nobody would dare to interfere. The idea, as I understood it, was that I would be nearby and take him quickly to my car.

Alejandro, when I told him this, smiled with appreciation of my father's plan. When I said I was surprised by what appeared to be at least a fleeting instance of strategic thinking, Alejandro said that he'd decided many months before not to be surprised by anything my father said that seemed to be ruled out by his condition or, more to the point, by the textbook expectations and predictions of the limited capacities of people who had been officially "assigned" to that condition. My father's absolute refusal to suppress whatever yearnings for autonomy remained to him, said Alejandro, no matter the problems it created for the staff—and no matter how upsetting it might be for us to see—was something to be celebrated, something to be seized upon as evidence of an unbreakable vitality.

Now and then, that restlessness exploded into language that was almost confrontational. "Can you take me with you now?" he asked one night in May when we were on the patio.

"Not now," I said.

"Yes! Now!"

His cheeks reddened. He clenched his fists and stared at me commandingly. He was the father. I was the son. He was not asking me for something this time. He was giving me instructions. As painful as this was to me, I relished his assertiveness.

On evenings when we stayed indoors, I would usually pull up a chair directly opposite the sofa where my father sat. Sometimes, however, he would make it obvious he wanted me to sit right next to him.

"Harry is over here," he told me once when I was sitting on the chair. When I got up and sat on the space beside him on the sofa, he took my wrist and lifted it and held it there in front of him and studied it a while.

"Who's holding it up?" he asked.

"You are, Daddy."

"No one else?"

"No one else. Only you."

He nodded at this. Then, with his left arm, he reached across my shoulder and drew me closer to his side, as if he wanted to believe he was protecting me.

"He sent you a letter not long ago," he said—although the last time he had written anything at all to me (it was not a letter, but another of those lists of annotations that Lucinda had sent on) had been nearly a year before—then spoke of "going to New York," which probably was suggested by the fact that I had told him of another trip I'd soon be making there.

He didn't ask if he could come with me, however. "I wish I could go with you," he said. "But I know I can't." A moment later, as if to explain why he was accepting this for now, he added, in a quiet voice, "I'm on the other side...."

Persnickety was lying on the floor across the room from us, pawing at the carpet underneath a coffee table and another sofa and noisily sniffing at something that excited her. When she became bored with this, she stood up and shook herself, a habit she had always had when she decided she'd exhausted all the possibilities of something that had captured her attention, then trotted back to sit before my father.

He didn't throw any cookies for her this time. He held her head and rubbed her ears and lightly touched the elevated area just above her nose.

"We have been so changed...," he said. I couldn't tell if he was speaking of Persnickety. He wasn't looking at her now. He was looking right at me.

"How much is left?" he asked.

I didn't try to answer. The question didn't seem to ask an answer. I stayed a while longer, until I saw that he'd begun to close his eyes.

His regular helpers were not there that night. A nurse came in to lift him from the sofa and bring him down the corridor and put him into bed. Outside, I gave Persnickety a chance to run in circles in the grass until she found a spot to please her. She squatted down and lifted her nose, as usual, as if she were studying the stars.

My father was ninety-five years old in August of 2001. My mother told me she would like to be with him to celebrate his birthday. I arranged for Silvia to bring her to the nursing home, since I had to be in Western Massachusetts earlier that day and would be arriving from the opposite direction.

They got there before I did. When they came in, Silvia said my father seemed a bit confused and somewhat distant and detached. But when my mother sat beside him and reached out one of her

61

hands to touch and gently graze his cheek, then placed it on his knee, he turned to her and said her name—"Ruth, darling…, Ruthie dear"—then lifted her hand and kissed her on her fingers many, many times.

Lucinda and Alejandro and his wife and two of the other people who'd been caring for my father were in the room as well. If I'm not mistaken, the teaching assistant who used to keep my parents company and help my father with his writing had come to visit too. There were also some people there who'd known my father long before his memory began to fail, and whom I didn't recognize, who came on their own. I had not invited them—it would never have occurred to me to do so. Besides, I thought the evening would be more relaxed, and less confusing for my father, if he were simply with my mother and Lucinda and the others he was close to.

It was a peculiar situation. I didn't know these people, although it's possible that they had once been closer to my father than I knew. I didn't want to disrespect them, but I felt their presence was invasive.

It did not turn out to be a comfortable evening. They sat around my father in a circle but spoke as if he were not there or couldn't hear what they were saying to each other. At one point, a woman who was sitting to the right side of the sofa raised her voice to speak across the room to me. "When the time comes, Jonathan," she said, "you know you can count on us. You're lucky to have had your father with you for so long. It's going to be hard for you to lose him. After the funeral...."

I cringed to hear her say this. She was sitting only a few feet from my father. Up until that moment, he'd been looking at his lap and did not appear to be attentive to the conversation. But, at those words, he suddenly looked up and said, not to the woman who had said this but to the room in general, "Is someone speaking of a funeral?"

The woman looked amazed to hear him say this. It was as if it now occurred to her, for the first time, that she had been speaking of a living person who was sitting there in front of her. But the damage had been done by then. I got up, went over to the sofa, and, touching my father's shoulder as he turned his eyes to me, I said to him, "Daddy, people say a lot of stupid things that they don't understand." They left shortly after that. He didn't seem to notice their departure.

My mother and the others stayed a while longer. When she left, she kissed my father on his forehead and she whispered, "Harry, darling...." In the car, as I drove her back into the city, I couldn't tell if she had been unsettled by that reference to a funeral. I was sure she'd heard the words, since the woman's voice had been so loud.

Lucinda later told me that she had been disturbed not only by the words themselves but by the way the visitors spoke "across" my father almost the entire time that they were there. I had noticed this as well. They were talking about Daddy as if he'd been reduced to a piece of silent stone that had no feelings and no possible awareness of what was taking place around him.

Lucinda also made the point that, on the few occasions when they did address themselves directly to my father, their voices had an artificial sound, as if they were engaging in some sort of ritual of pretended conversation. Many people talk this way when they are with Alzheimer's patients. Talking across them, rather than directly to them, is familiar too. I've heard a few physicians do this, speaking to me of my father's mental state—"loss of affect," "diminished capability to respond to stimuli"—while he was sitting there in front of us and looking at us quizzically.

"The thing of it is," Lucinda told me once, "I like to keep it real. I don't like having bullshit conversations with my patients that I'd never have with people outside of this building. I talk with your father, as much as I can, the same way that I like to talk with you and with my children and my friends. If I'm forced to bite my tongue and never tell him anything that feels authentic to me, I think it's degrading to his dignity. And, besides, it's boring. And the last thing that I want to do is bore a man who's known so many people who were obviously fascinating."

Like Silvia and Alejandro, she refused to dull my father's consciousness or underrate his possible responsiveness by speaking in placebos, and she never fell into that awful singsong tone, familiar in the nursery, that too many people use when they speak to patients who are elderly.

Lucinda was especially adept at eliciting those moments of sheer gaiety I have described when she was sparring with my father. In doing this, she brought the fresh air of the real world into his existence, driving out the grayness and the cognitive inertia that create a sense of semi-slumber in so many institutional environments. She loved to see the spark of life, and humor, and amusement, awaken in his eyes, which may be another reason why she had become incensed to hear somebody speak about his funeral in front of him.

Throughout that year, as in the years before, whenever Daddy made a reference, even the very briefest one, to something in his childhood, I would do my best to make an observation or to ask a question that I hoped might somehow stir a slightly deeper recollection of that memory.

I was convinced that, despite the seeming inaccessibility of many of these memories, and certainly his inability to put them into more than the most limited of verbal forms, my father had an inner life of cerebral activity—"a life beneath the life" is the way that I imagined this. One of the doctors whom I've questioned since my father's death spoke of this as an "oneiric" state, where memories, emotions, and diffuse ideas, although free-floating and amorphous in their nature, remain potentially "emergent properties" that might, at times, be activated by external stimuli or simply by spontaneous electrical events between the neurons in one or another portion of the brain.

I knew nothing of this at the time. But I was repeatedly persuaded, as when my father suddenly announced the members of his family, that there was a world of intermittent recollections, of memories or fragments of those memories, existing in a cloudy and anarchic kingdom of their own that might be summoned up "into the daylight," as it were, if I asked exactly the right question or struck upon a word or phrase that had an evocative association for him.

Not long, for instance, after he had made that reference to his parents and his sister and his brothers and had said his mother's name, "Rebecca," I made a calculated reference to his father, because he hadn't spoken of his father very much since he moved into the nursing home. As I've noted, Daddy called his father Pa. As soon as I asked him something about Pa, he smiled brightly and replied without a moment's hesitation, "He taught me how to sew...."

To any other person, at least to any person who did not know anything about my father's father, that answer might have seemed rather mysterious. But, right away, I knew exactly what he was referring to. As recently as 1993 or 1994, when he was living with my mother still, I had questioned him one night about his father's early years in the United States and he had answered in engrossing detail, even though my mother had to help him now and then to get the pieces of the story in the proper order. I took out a pad of paper and, when he noticed I was leaving sentences unfinished, because it wasn't easy to keep up with him, he would pause and then repeat himself.

He started by explaining that, although his father had arrived in Boston two years before his mother, he had not been able to succeed in his attempts to establish a financial foothold as a tailor and had been obliged to work instead in a sewing factory and, later, on a piecework basis, as a "presser," for example, in assisting other tailors. It was not until my grandma had arrived and begun to exercise her imposing power and to bring to bear her ingenuity in financial matters that my grandpa started his own tailor shop.

"He sat at a table and worked with an old machine that somebody had given him, which was operated by the pumping of a pedal. It was a Singer sewing machine. I remember it quite well because he took the time to teach me how to use it."

My grandma, by that time, had opened up the little store where she was selling milk and other groceries. Within a few more years, he said, "they had saved enough for Pa to turn the tailor shop into a clothing store." Daddy was twelve or thirteen now, and he remembered going after school to help out at the clothing store so his father could take off an hour, usually from four to five, to go home and have an early dinner, after which he would come back and work as late as nine. Sometimes, Daddy said, his mother also asked him to go in and help his father on the weekends.

His mother, he had mentioned, never asked this favor of his older brother, "whom she regarded as 'the scholar' in the family" and who, for this reason, was going to be spared any obligations that distracted from his studies. I asked if he had felt resentment of his mother's seeming favoritism for his brother. "You know Ma," he answered, not in a resentful tone but with a shrug of resignation. "No one in the family dared to argue with her."

Besides, he said, "I liked the clothing store, seeing all the working people coming in to buy those heavy boots and pants and sweaters that they needed for their jobs in the cold weather...." And, on weekends before holidays like Easter, "women from the neighborhood would crowd into the store looking for the pretty dresses and the stockings and especially the decorative hats" that were, he said, "an absolute necessity" for any kind of celebration in South Boston.

One Saturday, "two attractive women" came into the store who were "dressed provocatively." He didn't remember if his father had a fitting room but he said these women didn't seem to mind whether people saw them trying on a dress or undergarment right there in the middle of the store. "While Pa was fitting them, I watched very closely from behind a row of ladies' wear because I had never seen a woman's breasts exposed before." It was "quite a revelation" for an adolescent boy—and, he said, "more than an adequate reward" for giving up a Saturday to help out at the store.

Now, sitting in the nursing home, I had the brief temptation to make some passing mention of his father's store to see what other memories it might perhaps arouse. But Daddy's voice had trailed away after saying what he did about learning how to sew. And he was getting drowsy—it was nearly time for him to go to bed. Whatever else was brewing still within that "life beneath the life," floating somewhere in that dreamlike state, I had no way to know.

CHAPTER FIVE

Clinical Considerations: "All Tests Negative"

My father underwent a sudden crisis in his health in the autumn of 2001. It was the first time I was forced to face the possibility of losing him.

He had been having stomach difficulties of a mild nature for a week or more, until several days went by in which he passed no stool. Stomach problems of this kind, if not corrected promptly, are among the commonly precipitating causes of mortality in people of his age. Other familiar causes are infections of the urinary tract and swallowing and respiration difficulties. For this reason, vigilance in recognizing early warnings of these dangers is regarded as a matter of the highest order.

But the doctor who supervised the care of patients at the nursing home either wasn't made aware of my father's situation in a timely manner (his relationship to patients seemed to be quite indirect and, as Lucinda had confided in me, he was seldom there) or, knowing about it, chose to issue no instructions to the staff. For whichever of these reasons, the personnel on duty failed to make adjustments in my father's diet or administer a routine kind of enema before the problem grew severe. As a result, a blockage had developed in my father's rectum with an extensive backup into his large intestine.

I was in Seattle and Los Angeles that week. Lucinda was with her children on a holiday in Arizona. Alejandro also was away, and Silvia was preoccupied with funeral arrangements for one of her relatives. A new attendant, who was filling in for them, apparently did not have experience enough, or feel she had authority, to intervene.

When the medical director finally grew aware of how advanced the problem had become, he ordered an extreme and dangerous procedure in which a tube was forcibly inserted in my father's rectum and then as far as possible up into his colon.

My father, according to the temporary helper, "was screaming from the pain," but the person who was handling this instrument kept right on and thrust it into him more deeply. I was never able to find out from anyone responsible the sequence of events that followed next. It appeared, however, that the pain my father underwent, possibly compounded by damage to the lining of his colon from the penetration of the tube, had sent him into shock.

"The instrument they use for this," according to a doctor who explained this to me later, "is not only very long, twelve to sixteen inches typically, but it also has to be inflexible enough to break right through impacted stool, which can be as hard as stone, or get around the stool somehow to penetrate the colon. This is why procedures like this, which involve excruciating pain, need to be avoided.

"Well-trained doctors never use this method anymore. We teach our students to 'dis-impact' a patient's stool by hand, which does not incur the risk of causing a perforation of the colon and introducing an infection to the patient's bloodstream.

"In any event," he said, "so long as you monitor the patient very carefully, you shouldn't need to get into this situation. Especially for someone of your father's age, what he was subjected to was, frankly, inexcusable."

I was on the plane returning from Los Angeles on the day that all of this occurred. As soon as I landed, I found on my phone an urgent call from Silvia telling me to call the nursing home. When I did, someone at the nurses' desk told me that my father had been put into an ambulance, which, she believed, had taken him to Mount Auburn Hospital in Cambridge.

Upon arriving at the hospital, I was told that

he was in Intensive Care. Once I was identified as my father's son, one of the nurses brought me to his side.

I had never seen my father in a state like this before. His eyes were open, but his face was very pale. I leaned down close to him and spoke into his ear, and he looked up and seemed to try to speak; but he could not. When one of the residents took me aside to prepare me for the worst, I went out to the terrace of the hospital in order to decide if I should call my mother. I knew she'd want to see him if it became likely that he would not survive, but I didn't want to frighten her if I didn't need to. Instead, I tried to reach Lucinda but had no success— I didn't know at that time that she was away. With that exception, I remained there in the ICU or in a waiting room nearby. At some point after midnight I was told he had been stabilized and was no longer critical.

The following day I made up my mind to have him transferred to the MGH, which, as I realize now, was almost certainly unnecessary. I suppose I'd simply been conditioned by my father's long involvement with the MGH to believe that this must be the very best and safest place for him to stay while he was recovering.

In less than a week, he had returned to what physicians spoke of as his "baseline," a term employed to indicate his physical and mental state prior to the crisis he had undergone. At that point, I had to decide whether or not he should continue living at the nursing home.

In view of the apparent dereliction of the medical director, this was not an easy matter to resolve. It was only after talking with Silvia and Alejandro that I decided it would probably be best not to search around for another nursing home but to return him to a place that was familiar to him. I knew that Lucinda, now that she was back, would be looking after him with more than her usual attentiveness. I also knew that the companionship she gave him was not likely to be replicated in another institution, where no one on the staff would have her knowledge of his past experience and her understanding of his personality to draw upon in providing mental stimulation for him.

All in all, I think it was the right decision. The possibility, however, of a very different kind of alteration in the setting of my father's life would develop slowly in the months to come.

One afternoon a few weeks later, I opened up a number of the large sealed crates my father had insisted upon shipping to my house about twelve years before. Until this time, I had never felt the will to look into those boxes. Now, in the wake of the crisis he'd been through, I felt a sudden longing to immerse myself in whatever memories those packages might hold.

One of the crates I opened first contained a collection of notes and notebooks, case records and reports from his years in medical school and the years just following. Among these items, in an inexpensive frame, was my father's medical diploma. His day of graduation was June 21, 1934. In the same crate, also framed, was a certificate attesting to the period of time in which he'd done his internship at the MGH and stating he had "faithfully served as the East Medical House Officer in the Massachusetts General Hospital during the 19 months ending January 31, 1936." Under this certificate was a pile of file folders, held together by thick elastic bands, containing papers and case histories he'd written between 1936 and 1938, when he did two residencies, first at the Boston Psychopathic Hospital (now known as Massachusetts Mental Health), then at the Phipps Clinic of Johns Hopkins Hospital in Baltimore.

One of these papers, which I read with difficulty in his original handwritten version, was titled "A Case of Thalamic Syndrome Treated by Excision of a Cyst." The first section was the medical history my father had prepared, which described the patient, "a thin, frail, middle-aged woman," as having been admitted to the hospital "because she had complained of paroxysms of spontaneous pain" and "in hope of finding how much [of the] patient's pain is real or imaginary."

The patient, "the second of non-identical twins," my father had written, had been "a transverse presentation" and "was delivered after much manipulation and instrumentation." Following birth, "there was considerable delay and difficulty before breathing was established.... In 1900, at the age of five, she was seen at the Children's Hospital in Boston, where multiple contractures were observed on the left side of her body. Palliative surgical procedures were begun. Since the age of seven, there had been convulsive seizures, usually nocturnal....

"Examination of the cranial nerves" showed that "odors are poorly or not at all recognized through the left nostril. Vision is poor in the left eye.... There is atrophy and paresis [i.e., partial paralysis] of the left side of the face.... Hearing is diminished on the left. Taste on the left side of the tongue is less acute than on the right side, and at times is absent. Sensation on the left is also markedly abnormal. Once any sensation is produced, it is characterized by an unpleasant, at times painful quality.... There is no discrimination between sharp and dull objects.... A warm object is not described in thermal terms, but when ice is applied the patient screams that she is being 'burned.' "

He concluded that the pain of which the patient had complained was by no means imaginary. An electroencephalogram he administered two weeks later led him to believe there was a cyst on the right side of the woman's brain. A senior physician he called in for consultation believed that it had "almost certainly resulted from birth injury....A decision to operate was made after much discussion. The patient readily consented...."

The surgery, my father wrote, turned out to be successful ("since excision of the cyst..., patient has been free of sensory discomfort and has had no further seizures"), although he also noted adverse side effects and he appended several qualifications in speaking of the favorable outcome. "One's enthusiasm" for the procedure that had been undertaken should, he wrote, "be tempered" for these reasons.

Why did this material and the other cases in those file folders seize my fascination? The simplest reason, I suppose, is that they enabled me to follow my father in such a detailed way through several hundred hours of his work at a time, five months before I came into the world, when he was developing the clinical self-confidence as well as the cautious and self-critical capacities that won him the respect of the older doctors whom he looked on as his mentors. I noticed, for example, many phrases he'd crossed out, apparently because he felt that they were not sufficiently supported by the evidence of his examination. It was also obvious that he took a liking to the patient—"friendly and sociable..., an interesting raconteur..., she enjoyed conversations," a notation similar to many he would make in its appreciation of a patient's amiable qualities, if he thought the patient had such qualities, in case studies he would write for years to come.

Another set of documents, one I read with even greater interest, was a collection of my father's long summations of the cases of some thirty patients he had treated at Johns Hopkins, where he spent the following year on a Rockefeller grant under the direction of a Swiss-born psychiatrist, Dr. Adolf Meyer, who was one of the seminal figures in American psychiatry in the period when my father worked with him. (Dr. Meyer is generally credited by medical historians with having moved psychiatry in the United States "out of the asylum" and into the world of academic medicine.)

Under these summations, I discovered three large charts my father had made by pasting sheets of paper to a cardboard backing, each of which was three feet high and more than three feet wide, and which he'd apparently posted on his office wall to keep track of the progress of these patients. Each case had been described in eight sequential categories, starting with "Complaints and Symptoms," moving on to "Physical Findings," "Situational" and "Conditioning" factors, "Personality," "Heredity," "Treatment," and "Results and Follow-up"—all of which ran across the full length of the charts and under each of which he'd crammed as many details as the space would hold.

In one of the seemingly less complicated cases,

a woman, eighteen years of age, "hasty marriage, premarital pregnancy, difficult labor," had complained of a "choking feeling in [her] throat…, gasps for air, hands get numb, feels as if going to faint. Very much afraid." Under "Physical Findings," he had written, "Pt. is asthenic [i.e., of slender build] and underweight. Pulse 110. Reflexes ++. Blood pressure 125/60. E.E.G. negative." Under "Treatment": "Explain to pt. [that] physical findings [are] negative. Candid discussion w/ patient of probable causation. Anxiety attacks appear to be induced by fear of second pregnancy. Contraceptual diaphragm prescribed." Under "Results and Follow-up": "Uses diaphragm. No more numbness, choking sensation. No more fears. 'Not a single attack since….' Very happy now w/ husband."

In another case, that of a man twenty-seven years of age who had recently been fired from his job, "pt. suffers panic attacks, fear of death, palpitations, tingling [in] both arms, urge to defecate, profuse perspiration." Following his job loss, "sexual anxiety, insecurity. Pt. in love w/ woman in Florida, [but] fear of gonorrhea. Feels compulsion to escape, 'get up and get out of this relationship.'" Under "Treatment": "Discussion w/ pt. delineating factors precipitating [these] attacks. Explain etiology…." Under "Results and Follow-up": "Much improved. Fewer attacks." In a second follow-up, dated some months later:

"Affair in Florida going nicely. Expects to marry in one year...."

In one apparently more complicated case—a man forty-three years old "in business in Manila" who was suffering "constriction in [his] throat," "feeling of impending death," "anxiety attacks since 1928"—my father had asked Dr. Meyer to participate in the examination.

"Pt. describes attacks to Dr. Meyer: '[Feels] the way a man would feel if he had just fallen off a tall building. Terrified. Nothing can be done. You are finished. Just waiting to hit!'" Further along, my father noted, "Pt. raised by hysterical aunt.... Continually taken to doctors in [his] childhood. Lifelong hypochondriasis. Pt. indic.s castration fears...." Under "Heredity," he had written, "Paternal uncle: suicide. Father alcoholic. Mother carefree, luxury-loving, eloped w/ another man [and] deserted children. Pt. the youngest. One sister: beautiful, extravagant, married 3x...." My father's residency, it appeared, had come to an end before the case had been resolved. His last notation was the name of another doctor, perhaps another resident, to whom the patient's care had been assigned.

A neurologist in Boston to whom I later brought a number of these documents indicated that the emphasis and language in these clinical reports would in very few respects be regarded as archaic nowadays as a result of recent breakthroughs in our understanding of brain physiology. He also noted that the entries on these charts were of much historic interest because they reflected with fidelity the holistic theories for which Meyer was known and which incorporated "situational and social factors in the genesis of illness"—and not exclusively, or even primarily, episodes of trauma during childhood. These contemporaneous factors, he observed, were all too frequently dismissed by "rigid psychoanalysts" who were "blinded and dogmatic followers of Freud."

Perhaps, he said, one of the most important contributions that Meyer had made was his insistence upon highly detailed record keeping, which was not a common practice in American psychiatric institutions prior to his day. The diligence my father had invested in the preparation of those charts, which were so long they had been folded over several times in the first crate I had opened, set a pattern of exhaustive detail in the writing of case histories to which he would adhere for his entire career.

There were many far more personal items and idiosyncratic treasures buried in that crate. There were letters, for example, from people he had treated while he was a resident at the Boston Psychopathic who, upon recovery, had sent him notes of gratitude, apparently believing that a young physician less than two years out of medical school must deserve the credit for having worked "a miracle," rather than the more experienced physicians who were his superiors. Indeed, as early as 1931, when he was in medical school but was working part-time in the evenings at McLean, one of the patients he had helped to care for, a woman from Connecticut, wrote to ask if he'd have time to provide a "follow-up consultation" to her and her husband if they came up on the train to Boston! Attached to the letter by a rusted paper clip was the draft of a good-natured note in which my father had explained to her that he was only a medical student and not yet a doctor.

Incongruously packed into the midst of all of this was a pile of letters, tightly wrapped in a thick piece of cord, that my mother had written to my father while he was doing his internship at the MGH, as I gathered from the postmarks on the orange two-cent stamps that were on the corner of each envelope. I counted exactly fifty-one letters, which my mother had mailed to him every single day during a period when they were apart, except for one day when she sent two letters. I opened only three of them, feeling like a spy. They were love letters of a very tender and old-fashioned kind. Beneath the letters was a slender book of mischievously romantic poems by Edna St. Vincent Millay. I couldn't tell which of them had given it, or sent it, to the other.

In the subsequent weeks, whenever I had time, I gradually looked through several of the other boxes stored here at my house. Of all the items I discovered in these boxes, the one that awakened by far the most nostalgic memories was the old black doctor's bag my father carried with him when he was seeing patients at a hospital or sanatorium. The bag, which displayed all the signs of wear and tear one would expect from being used for all those years (patches of medical tape had been applied around the handles where the leather had peeled off), was still secured by a heavy metal clasp. My father had attached the key by a piece of wire when he sent it to me.

There was nothing unusual about the contents of the bag. I found an old blood-pressure gauge with an inflatable purple band attached, neatly folded in a dark blue case, a stack of about a dozen wooden throat sticks held together by elastics, a box of Band-Aids, sterile dressing sponges, packages of alcohol wipes, a metal reflex hammer with a rubber head, and a two-pronged metal fork, resembling a tuning fork about six inches long, that was used to test a patient's hearing by holding it first at a distance from the ear, then moving it closer by small degrees until the patient heard it. There was also an impressive-looking Fleischer stethoscope with the name of the manufacturer, "Dickinson and Co.," printed on the back side of the metal piece my father placed against a patient's chest.

When I took out that stethoscope and held it in my hands, a memory I'd long forgotten came into my mind of a time when I was very young, not more than six or seven, and my father on an impulse took me with him to McLean one night when the resident on duty called him at our home to tell him that one of his patients had become unusually distraught and was talking about suicide. I remember he had just come home and begun to have his dinner, and, as usual when a call for him came in at night, my mother put her hand across the mouthpiece of the phone and asked him, "Harry, are you here?" And, as almost always, my father nodded yes to her and got up to take the call.

A moment later, his dinner was forgotten. He plunked me down beside him in his car, my mother watching from the doorway, and before long we were far away in Belmont (it seemed like far away to me), going up the driveway to the hospital.

My father had a likable and, I would guess, somewhat unconventional way of initiating conversations with his patients. He spoke, from the start, with a friendly informality. He joked with his patients. He could make them laugh sometimes even when they felt they had been drowning in depression or anxiety. So it probably did not surprise a patient, or the nurses at a hospital, when he showed up now and then with his son in tow.

In any case, he said to the patient, "You are going to be examined first"—or something to the same effect—"by my chief assistant." Then he lifted me up and put me on the bed and handed me the stethoscope and put the black plugs in my ears and showed me where to hold the metal disk against the patient's chest. I listened as carefully as I could and probably tried to give a knowledgeable look, as children will do when they've been placed for a moment or two in a position that seems terribly important. While I was doing this, my father was studying the patient's hands and eyes and his expression. Then he took the stethoscope and began to give the man a full examination. That's all I remember.

The reason I was looking at the stethoscope so closely, and holding it so carefully, was that I was thinking of how many times—thousands of times, I suppose—he must have put those plugs into his ears and listened to the heartbeats and the respiration of his patients, doing what his training as a doctor taught him he must do even before he began to ask the probing questions he had learned to ask as a psychiatrist. But I was also thinking of how many nights my father had to get up from his dinner because emergencies like this came up so often and because he'd grow uneasy, and feel negligent, if he remained there at the table while a patient was disconsolate.

Most nights, naturally, when these calls came in, he would not impulsively decide to bring me with him. He would simply leave us there and head straight for the door. If I wasn't sleeping deeply, I might hear him when he got home late at night and might hear my mother talking with him as she heated up his dinner.

I know the time has long since passed when doctors, no matter what their specialty might be, would interrupt their private lives so willingly in order to fulfill their sense of obligation to a patient. Maybe it's beyond all reason to regret the passing of that era. Still, I wished the doctor at the nursing home had retained a little more of that tradition of attentiveness. I would come to have the same wish later on about another geriatrician my father would rely upon. I never felt they gave him back in full, or even in small part, what he had given once unstintingly to people who had placed their trust in him.

One further memory, which holds less personal significance for me but which I find intriguing as a kind of window into the psychiatric world of Boston more than half a century ago, will come here as a sidenote to a longer story I have touched upon already. In one of the crates that contained some legal documents pertaining to Eugene O'Neill, I found a folder of remarkable materials about a confrontation into which my father had been drawn with one of his longtime friends and colleagues, a psychiatrist named Merrill Moore, who had grown involved with the O'Neills before O'Neill became my father's patient.

Moore was one of Boston's preeminent psychiatrists and also was a literary person with close associations in the world of theater. He had been selected to examine the playwright's wife, Carlotta, at a time when she herself was ill—the initial diagnosis had identified her illness as "hysteria"—and had been transported to McLean. Moore had been retained, as I discovered now, by a close acquaintance of O'Neill, the prominent New York producer Lawrence Langner, who was also a director of the Theatre Guild. But Moore had managed to mishandle the case in a way that did a grave injustice to Carlotta.

Dr. Moore, to whom my father introduced me once years later at the Harvard Club in Boston, was a brilliant man but also widely viewed as a lovable eccentric. He wrote poetry—sonnets exclusively, and apparently in great profusion (several thousand, as he claimed), which he was more than willing to recite to friends and patients. For a time, he liked to carry bean seeds in his pocket and would hand them out to people in a jovial manner. "Harry," he once said when he shook hands with my father, "plant these in your garden," and he left a couple bean seeds in my father's palm, for which my father thanked him in good humor.

The problem, however, according to my father, was that Moore, for all of his unquestioned psychiatric expertise, had been perfunctory and hasty in his observation of Carlotta and had overlooked the fact that what appeared to be psychosis was actually the temporary consequence of bromides she'd been taking in excessive doses. Even after he had been alerted to her bromide poisoning, he continued to dismiss it as the reason for her illness. Instead, he insisted that she was psychotic and told officials at McLean that he intended to declare her "legally insane." He further recommended that the playwright and his wife should permanently separate. It appeared that he had come to this conclusion before he had examined her.

Both Carlotta and O'Neill would later suffer greatly for this misguided intervention, because O'Neill had been sufficiently unwise as to acquiesce at first in Dr. Moore's advice and agreed to sign a paper, known as a "petition," prepared by a lawyer in New York and cosigned by Dr. Moore, alleging that she was insane and incapable of managing her own affairs. Carlotta never forgave her husband for this "act of treachery," as she would refer to it repeatedly.

By this time, in any case, officials at McLean became alarmed at Dr. Moore's intention to arrange a permanent commitment for Carlotta—"involuntary mental hospitalization" was the term—which they considered medically unjustifiable. My father was asked to enter the case, examine Carlotta neurologically as well as psychiatrically, and present them with a diagnosis, as he'd done for other patients at McLean over a period of years. My father did the examination, as requested, and concluded that Carlotta was most definitely not insane and therefore not committable.

When this information was relayed to Moore, his response was adversarial. "One day in April," my father wrote in a long and detailed memo, "I got a telephone call from Merrill Moore. He said that he was in New York" and that he "and some of the playwright's friends," whom he did not name, were convinced that *both* Carlotta and O'Neill were legally insane, that their marriage ought to be dissolved, and that separate guardianships should be established. In the playwright's case, his affairs would then be handled by a group of people in New York, presumably the people who believed he was insane, who would make decisions, for example, on the uses of his literary properties.

In spite of my father's affectionate relationship with Dr. Moore, his behavior in this instance struck my father as not only unprofessional but legally quite dangerous. He said he was compelled to challenge him directly.

"I crackled out the following: 'Your patient [meaning O'Neill, whom Daddy had not yet examined] may be crazy. Mine is not. I'll have nothing to do with such a scheme,'" and, he added, he'd do everything he could "to frustrate and prevent it." When Moore persisted, Daddy said, "Merrill, are you out of your mind?" And he cautioned him that he was being drawn into a situation that might be regarded by a legal body as "a criminal conspiracy." Moore, he wrote, "sort of backed off," and the conversation ended.

Shortly thereafter, my father was approached by one of O'Neill's most trusted friends, a powerful theatrical figure and level-headed man named Russel Crouse, who asked if he would travel to New York to talk directly with O'Neill and try to provide whatever help he could in clearing up the medical morass and personal misunderstandings Moore had left behind. At the request of Mr. Crouse, my father also gave O'Neill the kind of classic psychiatric interview and neurological examination he had given to Carlotta.

He came to the conclusion that, while psychiatric factors and the maddening obstruction of his creative powers by his physical debilitation obviously played a major role in his unhappiness, O'Neill was clearly not insane from any medical or legal point of view. His right to make his own decisions, even if decisions he might make were to be affected to a large degree by the strong will and protective judgment of his wife, could not be taken from him.

During the course of this examination, O'Neill made it apparent that he now regretted having given in to Dr. Moore's advice and that he wanted to be reunited with his wife. I don't know the rest of this—my father's notes are incomplete, or there may be others I have yet to find. But I gather that O'Neill found something that he liked and trusted in the way my father spoke with him and questioned him and, as I've said, there seemed to be a comfortable rapport between the two of them. This is a long way of explaining in more detail than before the somewhat convoluted pattern of events that led O'Neill to ask my father to become his doctor.

Carlotta, meanwhile, who had left McLean about a month before, now made arrangements for a suite of rooms that overlooked the river in the small but very nice hotel opposite my father's office. My father met O'Neill when he arrived at Back Bay Station with a nurse who had traveled with him from New York, and brought him to Carlotta, who treated him, at least at first, forgivingly and lovingly. Although they would have bitter quarrels, which, according to my father, had been a pattern in their lives for many years, the final truth, in his belief, is that the two of them were totally dependent on each other.

O'Neill told my father that, for all the miseries they underwent together and the many cruelties they never ceased inflicting on each other, he could not live without Carlotta and he knew she would protect him and his interests, as she had done with fierceness and fidelity throughout the decades of his greatest productivity. And, certainly, in terms of his physical well-being during the time when he was in my father's care, she did protect him patiently and tirelessly, following instructions that my father gave her, phoning him repeatedly when she thought that there might be a reason for concern.

Sometimes, too, she would call my father, at

O'Neill's request, on an evening, often very late, when O'Neill became unusually depressed and told her he'd feel better if he had a chance "to talk with Harry" for a while. The sight of my father rushing in and taking out his stethoscope to do a quick check of his vital signs, and then remaining there to chat with him for ten or fifteen minutes before he went to bed, apparently provided him with a sense of reassurance that enabled him to get to sleep more easily.

As my mother had explained to me, my father didn't like the mediating role in which he was often placed when Carlotta and O'Neill were at odds with one another, and I have described his discontent at being placed by other families in a similarly difficult position. In all of his cases, nonetheless, whether those involving people who were privileged and famous or those of the very poor or marginally middle class to whom he attended for long periods of his career, he never ceased to be the medical doctor he'd been trained to be. The old black doctor's bag accompanied him everywhere.

CHAPTER SIX

A Sentimental Longing

Throughout the end of autumn and the winter of 2001, and well into the spring and summer of 2002, Daddy kept on asking whether it was time yet for me to take him home—whether to my mother's home or to my own was never really clear. Or sometimes, as we've seen, he would simply ask me whether he could come with me *wherever* I was going when he saw me getting up to leave. The wistfulness with which he asked these questions brought back to me a memory from nearly sixty years before.

When I was a child around the age of seven my mother and father sent me to a summer camp in Maine. They had been uncertain whether I was old enough to be away from home, but Daddy had decided that it would be good for me to see if I could overcome my shyness and manage for a short time on my own. He was also confident that making friends with the other campers and getting caught up in the camp's activities, like "color wars," which were a familiar part of summer camp for children in those days, would probably distract me from missing him and my mother quite as badly as my mother feared. He discovered quickly he was wrong.

"The letters you sent us were universally unhappy. They ranged from pitiful to plaintive. 'When are you going to come to visit? When are you going to take me home?'" But, he said, "every time we got in the car and drove up to the camp—we must have done this several times, because your letters were like little masterpieces of unqualified despair— you would look amazed and you would want to know what we were doing there." So, after talking with some of the counselors or the camp director, "your mother and I would feel relieved and we'd go back to Boston." But then, he said, "as soon as we got home, there would be another letter, even sadder than the one before!

"I think, in the end, we brought you home before the session ended. Those letters of yours, which you must have written almost every day, were too much for us to bear...."

That was in 1943 or 1944. I could still remember going up the steps to the camp director's office every afternoon to buy another postage stamp so I could tell my parents just how horrible it was that they had abandoned me. Now my father was the child and I was the grown-up he depended on. And this time it was he who kept on asking how much longer it would be before I brought him home.

There were also times, of course, when I would arrive and he would appear to be entirely caught up in the company of Silvia or Alejandro or Lucinda and I would, maybe for the first few minutes, feel as if my presence was almost superfluous. That didn't last long, however, and when it was time for me to leave, even if he didn't ask if he could come with me, my father's eyes would follow me as I was heading for my car.

I could not take my father home with me, not to the small and isolated village where I had been living. I did wonder now and then whether there was any way at all, if I put a very solid system of support in place, that he might be able to return to the apartment where he had been living with my mother up until six years before. His needs, however, were so great, and the questions of logistics I would have to face seemed so complex—if any plan like this were even feasible in medical respects—that I would promptly put it out of mind. It would return, a lingering thought, a kind of daydream, off and on; but, as much as his repeated pleas would sadden me and tear at me, the whole idea remained within a realm of the implausible.

Then one evening in the end of winter—it was late in March 2002—I mentioned this to Silvia. To my surprise, she said that she had recently begun to have the same thoughts too. "You know," she said, "he's always asking the same question now. 'Is it time yet to go home?'" Selecting her words carefully, because she didn't want to seem presumptuous, she said that she'd begun to wonder if he really needed to remain here any longer. "If you want to bring him home to live there with your mother, I think I could care for him if I had some other people I could count on to take turns with me."

I was grateful for her offer, but I told her I would need to think about it more and would want to talk with Alejandro and Lucinda. I also wondered if I ought to bring it up with my father's trust attorney, since he shared with me, theoretically at least, some responsibility for decision making for my father.

I turned first to Alejandro, who had observed my father closely now for several years. I didn't ask him, at this point, about the medical considerations that would have to be addressed or about the question of arrangements for my father's care that Silvia had raised. There was a different question in my mind—one that I already sensed would be the hardest to resolve.

Alejandro was, of course, familiar with my father's frequent voicing of his wish, or at times almost peremptory demand, to be permitted to "go home." What I didn't know, however, was the way it might affect him to return, no matter how much he insisted that he wanted this, to a place he hadn't seen for several years and which, I thought, he might not even recognize to be his "home" at all.

Even though there was a beautiful apartment in a high-rise building, with a view of the Charles River and the Cambridge skyline, in which he had lived for more than twenty years, and even though the handsome desk at which he'd worked for most of his career remained there by one of the windows with his pads of paper and manila folders and his medical desk references exactly where they'd been before, what meaning would this place, this desk, and all the objects it contained, not even to speak of my mother's presence in the same apartment, hold for him at this stage of his illness? In this respect, I had to ask myself, *was* there a home in any sense— would there ever be a home again—my father could return to?

Alejandro told me he'd been thinking for a while now about the possibility that I'd discussed with Silvia. But he also said he'd asked himself a question not unlike the one that I had posed.

"Does he yearn for something," Alejandro asked, "that may turn out, in the limits of his recognition and his consciousness, to be no longer 'there'?" He also said he had to wonder whether we could ever know for sure if this apartment, this specific place in Boston, was, in fact, the home that he was thinking of. "Your father has spoken to me many times about his mother and the building in South Boston where he lived when he was a boy," and it had been only a couple years before that my father had imagined he was having conversations with his mother on the phone. Which home, which place, which potential destination, Alejandro asked, was my father yearning for?

"Then too," he said after a bit of hesitation, "'going home' might have another, very different meaning for him. Something different altogether...."

It was April when I had this talk with Alejandro. Soon after that, I had a longer talk about this with Lucinda. In answer to the question I'd discussed with Alejandro, she said she found it very hard to guess the way it might affect my father to return to his apartment. But, because she'd come to be a close friend to my mother in the visits she had made to the apartment, she introduced a wholly separate question that I hadn't really thought about before.

She told me she recognized, from her conversations with my mother, that beneath the sense of loss and sadness she had undergone when my father moved into the nursing home, there were also complicating factors in my mother's state of mind that led her to find his absence from their home—"awful as it sounds!" Lucinda said—"a great relief to her." One of those factors, which may come as no surprise to people who have lived with family members who were going through the early stages of dementia, had been a periodic series of events in which his growing restlessness would suddenly erupt into a loss of emotional control that had alarmed her greatly.

More than once, my father had flailed out at her after something none too sensitive that she had said about his growing loss of competence in dealing with financial matters—tearing up bills, for instance, that he incorrectly thought he had already paid and writing intemperate letters to the companies that sent them.

My mother had a sharp tongue when she grew impatient with my father, and she didn't seem to recognize how easily her comments could reduce him to humiliation. At one of those times he pushed her away from him abruptly and she lost her balance and landed on the hardwood floor next to the bedroom door.

As soon as he saw what he had done, my father got down on the floor, put his arms around my mother's body, and apologized abjectly. Later, in the nursing home, he wrote her some remorseful letters making clear that he had not forgotten this or, if not this actual event, that he at least retained a memory of having done some things that had been harmful to her.

"Dear Ruth," he said in one of these letters, which was written soon after he had gone into the nursing home, "I hope you will discard any unpleasant memories that you may have and will shortly feel much better. I look forward to a most agreeable resolution of misunderstandings that have come between us. Looking forward to uniting with you promptly...."

A second letter, written a year later: "This is by Harry L. Kozol M.D. as a giant apology to my beloved wife Ruth M. Kozol. I can never stop loving you and never shall. I shall try to make up for whatever harm I may have done you...."

The last of several letters that he sent my mother, this one also written in the second year after he had moved from the apartment, did not express apologies for "whatever harm" he'd done, which it's likely he no longer could recall, but simply conveyed a longing for my mother and a sense of urgency about returning to their home. "My dearest beloved wife residing at 780 Boylston Street, Boston, Mass. Today is Wednesday. I hope to return to the loving companionship of my desperately needed wife. I BEG OF YOU. PLEASE HELP ME!"

I don't think I'd seen these letters when my father wrote them. As best I can recall, Lucinda had not shown them to me. They were my father's letters to my mother, not to me, and it may be that, in her sensitivity, she was trying to respect this small degree of privacy between them.

My mother, according to Lucinda, who brought the letters with her when she went to the apartment, was obviously moved and spoke with kindness and compassion of my father. But her recollection of his turbulent behavior and, as she told Lucinda, other moments when she'd had the feeling he was on the verge of reaching out and striking her, had left her, understandably, with a degree of fear that may not have wholly dissipated with the years.

Once he was in the nursing home, those episodes of physical unruliness came under reasonable, if incomplete, control, in part because of anti-anxiety medication he received. Still, his restlessness resurfaced periodically and, once his injured hip had healed and he could stand and walk without assistance, it became self-evident that he needed careful supervision on the part of his attendants or, late at night when they weren't there, the regular staff workers. There was the ever-present risk that he might do himself real harm if he should awaken in the middle of the night, manage to get out of bed, and walk into a door or wander out into the hall.

Misadventures of this sort had taken place a number of times when staff members were distracted by emergencies or, as happened more often than it should, were caught up in their purely social conversations at a distance from his room. Once he walked into a rack of medication trays that was directly in his path. Another time, he walked into a female patient's room, which eventuated in no harm to her, or to himself, but elicited her outraged squeals. (I admit I was amused by Lucinda's characteristically irreverent observation: "I think she was delighted by the scandalous idea that a man your father's age might find her irresistible!")

Even in the most recent years, moreover, as the increasing weakness of his legs prevented him from walking any distance on his own, my father still was able, if by inadvertence the guardrail of his bed had not been raised, to climb out of bed and wander around a little in his room until he bumped into a chair or, in one instance, fell down on the floor.

When I brought these matters up with Alejandro in a second conversation later in the spring, he dispelled them rapidly. "Your father's physical turbulence is not an issue anymore. He represents no danger to your mother or to anybody other than himself." The physical precautions taken in the nursing home to guarantee his safety were, in any case, "not especially impressive," Alejandro noted, and could easily be duplicated, and made more consistent, by attendants such as Silvia who might care for him at home.

The medical supervision by the doctor at the nursing home was, as both of us had seen, more or less a fiction. "He comes in and looks at patients' records, maybe writes prescriptions, issues some instructions....I don't know how frequently, if ever, he conducts examinations." A good arrangement with a doctor I might find in Boston would, he thought, be likely to provide much better supervision. Lucinda, as he noted, was one of the few members of the staff who gave my father thoroughgoing medical attention. Perhaps, he said, there might be a way that she could keep on seeing him, maybe on a weekly basis, if in fact I did decide at last to bring him home.

There was a final question in my mind, however, which I did not share with Alejandro. Even without the slightest risk of danger to my mother's safety, I had to wonder what effects the plan I was considering might have upon the well-established patterns of accommodation she had made to living in his absence.

Without being disrespectful to my mother, who was holding up with a good deal of courage in the face of a variety of small infirmities, including some arthritic pains, and the normal loss of energy in someone who was nearly ninety-nine years old, it is only honest to concede that she had grown increasingly tyrannical in her reliance on the constant presence of the people who looked after her. Even with the slightly larger team of helpers Silvia believed that she could put together to take care of both of them at once, I didn't have the least idea of how my mother would react to sharing their attention with my father.

It was time for me to go and have a conversation with my mother.

The apartment where my parents had been living since they moved into the city in the early 1970s consisted of a good-size bedroom, a second bedroom where the people caring for my mother could lie down and get some rest once she'd gone to sleep, and a large, attractive living room, at one end of which my father's desk remained the centerpiece and at the other end of which there was a dining area and, just adjacent to the dining area, a small and narrow kitchen.

My mother still could walk into the living room, usually on her own, or with some assistance from her helpers. In good weather they would sometimes bring her downstairs to the mezzanine of the apartment building, which opened on a grassy area where she could enjoy the sun and see young people strolling by and walk along the flower beds and hedges on the far side of the lawn.

When it was too cold to go outside, her helpers walked with her along the corridors or in the lobby area every afternoon, after which she liked her daily ritual of having tea and English biscuits at the dinner table, where her helpers usually would sit and join her.

At night, during the baseball season, she liked to watch the Red Sox games. Before my father's accident, they often used to watch the ball games on a large screen at the Harvard Club and would sometimes have dessert or dinner there. My father liked to pick up conversations with people he had never met before, graduate students, lawyers or physicians, other academic people, mostly of my generation, whom my mother said that both of them found more interesting to be with than the rapidly diminishing number of their peers.

Now, in the evenings, my mother would sit up in bed to watch the games. I had given her a Red Sox jersey as a birthday present when she was ninety-five. Her helpers said she liked to wear it, as a good luck symbol, while she cheered for players whom she recognized from long familiarity. In earlier years she had been a fan of Roger Clemens. But when Clemens ended up pitching for New York, her opinion of him quickly changed. "He's gotten too fat. We're better off without him." (Before long, she replaced him in her loyalties with Pedro Martinez.) A few years later, when the Red Sox finally broke their famous curse and brought home a championship after more than eighty years, my mother was triumphant.

I asked her once if she recalled the previous time the Red Sox had brought home a victory. She could not remember exactly in what year it was but she said, "I was a teenager then. I was at Girls' Latin School"—a highly respected secondary school that has, however, since been closed. She said she'd never seen a game until she was older, because she had to study hard to keep up with the rigorous curriculum for which her school was famous. In addition to this, three afternoons a week, she had to take the trolley train from her home in Dorchester all the way to Symphony Hall, where one of the violinists of the Boston Symphony, who was acquainted with her mother, had been giving her instruction since the age of ten on a violin that she had saved for all these years, still in the old and tattered case she carried on the trolley.

When there was no ball game or when it came on too late because the team was playing in the west, she usually stayed up long enough to watch the TV news at ten. Then the person taking care of her would lower the reclining bed and stay there in the room with her until she fell asleep.

Among her helpers at the time, the one to whom she felt the closest and who had cared for her the longest was a woman of about my age whose name is Julia Walker and whose children I had known when I was teaching in her neighborhood in the 1960s. Julia told me recently that, up until the age of ninety-nine, my mother insisted upon looking at the Boston Globe each afternoon or evening. When the gradual impairment of her reading vision made it hard for her to do this, Julia would pick out a few important stories and would read them to her, and discuss them with her—political stories for the most part, Julia said, that she knew would be of interest to my mother.

My mother, who had been an unrelenting liberal as long as I recalled, remained attuned to politics, although she grew amusingly confused when George W. Bush was elected president in November 2000. "We already *had* him long ago!" she said to Julia, mixing up Bush the father with the son. "What's he doing back again?"

I don't want to overstate my mother's clarity of thinking. Now and then she'd make an observation about somebody in public life that had, at best, a very tenuous and whimsical connection to reality. "Hillary Clinton is sick of being married to her husband," she announced to me and Julia one night in 2001. "She's ready to get rid of him."

"I wouldn't be surprised," said Julia, "after what he's put her through."

"I think she wants to marry Jonathan," my mother said.

"Why *me*?" I asked.

Julia looked at me with sympathy.

But my mother kept right on. "She isn't getting enough attention from her husband. She needs to get remarried." That, to my relief, was her final word for now on what would come to be one of her favorite subjects of discussion.

Apart from this maternal fantasy and a couple others that she found appealing and allowed herself to entertain from time to time, my mother's thinking had continued to be reasonably clear. The attorney who was managing my father's trust and hers believed she was still competent to sign her income tax returns, which she did with the attorney's pen in an only slightly shaky hand. Like my father, she had appointed me to be her healthcare proxy in anticipation of a time when she would no longer have the judgment to arrive at an informed decision in a medical emergency. That time had not yet come, however, and I had no wish to limit her autonomy in this or any other area in which she chose to exercise her will and make her own decisions.

A handful of people who had visited my mother after Daddy went into the nursing home had rather briskly written off her competence because, when they arrived at the apartment, she would pretty much ignore them and, more than once, she actually refused to speak with them. On one of these visits, after keeping silent for a while, she flatly said, "I don't trust you. I don't want to talk to you. Go home!"

Their natural reaction was to reaffirm the uninformed assumption they'd already made prior to their visits: a self-confirming process since my mother recognized the way they looked upon her and, I thought, was fighting justifiably in defense of her own dignity when she wouldn't let them lead her into conversations that were obviously intended to be tests of her lucidity.

One of them said to me, "She's crazy as a loon! She wouldn't even talk to me!" I didn't think that this was crazy in the least. She loved to talk at length with Julia and Lucinda, and with several of my younger friends who were very fond of her and had known her long before my father became ill. Why did she look forward to the time they spent with her and talk with them so openly? I think it was because she knew that they respected her.

Even on those evenings when she yielded to her fantasies, there was always something faintly comical about her tone of voice, which, no matter how positive or stubborn she might sound, seemed to signal that she knew she might be wandering into a region of the only semi-real. "I think your mother knows deep down when she's 'stretching' something that she'd kind of like into a reality," said Julia. "I think she knows the difference. It's like something that she plays with for a while. If I tell her I think she's incorrect in something that she's said, it always seems to slow her down or bring the story to an end." That was my experience as well. It didn't often take more than a few no-fooling words to bring my mother back into the world of actualities.

As late as in the previous fall, she still retained sufficient rationality and independence in her thinking to make a major medical decision without asking my approval or opinion. Her physician had detected something that he found irregular, and worrisome, in one of my mother's ovaries. A biopsy revealed a cancerous growth—but small and highly localized.

The doctor, who was not a geriatrician but was widely known in Boston as an excellent practitioner, talked with me about the risks a woman of her age would inevitably face even in a fairly routine surgical procedure. The likelihood that she'd come out of this without complications was, he told me, relatively good. "She's got a lot of spunkiness and fire in her still....If you decide you want to go ahead, I'll make the referral and we'll put her in the MGH. I'd like to get it done as fast as possible."

My mother, when I spoke to her about this, said that she'd already made her own decision. "Go ahead! Get it done! I don't want to die yet. I'll *tell* you when I'm ready...."

I put her into Phillips House, a section of the MGH in which a little more than the usual attention could be given to a patient. She underwent the various preoperative procedures, went into surgery on a Monday morning, emerged from anesthesia safely, and was kept in the hospital for only three more days before they sent her home to her apartment, where she made a fairly swift recovery.

This, then, was the background for the conversation with my mother that I had put off, longer than I should, about the plan I had been contemplating for my father.

On an evening late in June, I sat beside my mother's bed and told her what I had been thinking about Daddy. I summarized the medical issues I'd discussed with Alejandro. I told her of the offer Silvia had made. I also told her that I had no way to know, and nobody I'd talked with seemed to know, how it would affect my father to come back and live in the apartment.

In spite of his apparent stamina, I said, no one could predict how much longer he would live. He might live for several years; but I also knew a single bout of serious infection or problems that might come up in a surgical procedure, if for any reason that should be required, could easily put him in a critical condition from which he would not emerge. Before this happened, as I tried my best to explain this to my mother, I had the strongest yearning—and I told her that I knew it might be unrealistic—to let my father live his final days at home.

She didn't let me go on any further with my explanations. "I want him to come home," she said.

I insisted upon pressing her about the possibly disruptive changes this would bring into the pattern of her life. My father's needs, as I reminded her, were greater than her own. How did she feel about the fact that, with my father living here, she would likely not receive as much attention from the people taking care of them as she was receiving now?

"I want him to come home," she said again, dispensing with my question. "Your father's like a child now. He's been away from home too long. Go and buy a bed for him. Buy whatever else he needs. Tell the lawyer to write me a check."

I told her I'd been thinking that I ought to ask the lawyer for advice before proceeding with these plans.

"Why waste time with *him*?" she said. "Tell him I've made up my mind. I don't need to ask for his permission. He's a lawyer—slow as molasses! I've made my decision."

I asked her, if we were to do this, whether she would want me to put Daddy's bed—he would need a hospital bed—here beside her in her bedroom or in the other bedroom. Her answer wasn't sentimental in the least. "Why would I want him in this room? I'd never get a chance to sleep. Put him in the other room. Set up another bed for Julia out there in the living room."

I still had questions in my mind, but she didn't want to hear them. She had thought this through as much as she intended to.

"Don't talk about it to me anymore! Go tell Julia that I'd like a cup of tea. We'll have it in the dining room."

So that was the end of our discussion about Daddy. I went out to share the news with Julia. She knew what I'd been thinking. Silvia, whose polite but uncontainable take-over inclinations had already set themselves in motion, had, of course, shared her thoughts with Julia. So the only news that I was giving Julia was the way my mother had reacted and her insistence that I shouldn't talk about it anymore.

"She gives you a hard time," Julia said. "Bless her, that's your mother!"

Julia and I took out the box of biscuits that my mother liked and cut up some pieces of Camembert and Emmenthal and brought them to the table. I got out my mother's favorite teapot and we had our tea, the three of us, as usual, together. My mother's cranky attitude had disappeared as quickly as it had begun. As soon as we were finished, I got up and kissed her and made my escape before she had a chance to get annoyed with me again.

The only disapproving comment that she managed to get in was a reference to the slightly shabby-looking sweater I was wearing.

"Do me a favor. Go and buy yourself a decent sweater. Go next door to Lord and Taylor. Please don't skimp on something cheap."

I didn't actually need a sweater. I already had two extra sweaters she had given me that I'd never worn. But I promised her I'd do this anyway. I wanted to get out that door and have a chance to do some quiet thinking on the drive back to my home. In spite of the explicit orders she had handed down, it would be a while more before I could arrive at a decision.

CHAPTER SEVEN

Coming Home

In the months that followed, while I wrestled with my last remaining reservations about giving notice to the nursing home, Silvia and Alejandro and the others who filled in for them continued to spend pleasant afternoons and evenings with my father. As often as I could, I would drive down to be with him in the early evening.

The weather in the end of June was already summerlike, and there was a period of almost torrid weather in the first weeks of July. In the village where I lived, teenage boys and older men brought their fishing lines and tackle boxes to the edges of a rushing stream that ran right through the center of the town. They'd usually go down there as the heavy branches of the trees were starting to cast shadows on the water and would stay until the sun went down.

One evening, sitting with my father on the patio, I told him that I'd seen a group of boys that afternoon fishing from a rocky ledge a quarter mile from my home. I told him it reminded me of when he used to take me fishing with him on a lake in Maine when I was a child, maybe eight or ten years old. I lifted my arms and swung a long imaginary rod to imitate a cast and he copied me, swinging his arms together in an arc the way that he had taught me.

I realized that there may have been no memory involved in this at all. It may have been no more than an automatic imitation of the motion I had made. But his eyes had brightened and, even though he didn't speak a word that might have indicated any kind of recollection, he made that casting motion several times, looking out beyond the wooden railing of the patio as if to see the spot on which the plug had landed.

Everything about those fishing trips had been a great adventure for me—the darkness of the deep pine forests, the stillness of the water when we went down to the dock and made our preparations. We'd usually rent a rowboat with an outboard motor so we could cross the wide and open section of the lake. Then we'd turn the motor off and use the oars to get into one of those isolated coves where the fish were feeding in the early morning. We would take turns standing in the bow and trying to cast into a darkened spot as close as possible to shore. As often as not, the lure would get stuck on a piece of wood beneath the surface or a snatch of lily pads and we'd have to move the boat and reach our hands as far down into the water as we could to try to free the lure. If we couldn't free it, we'd have to cut the line and attach another lure and begin all over.

My father had all kinds of lures with brightly colored feathered tails, and narrow filaments made from catgut, I believe, to attach them to the fishing line, and a big curved fisherman's knife, and cans of oily substances with narrow spouts, each in its own small subdivided space within the tackle box. I still had that tackle box and two long rods with beautiful reels, marbled-looking on their sides, stored in my garage. When I had opened the tackle box a month or so before, the odor of oils and the other smells that it released brought back a flood of memories.

I had thought of bringing it with me someday to the nursing home, wondering if those silver spoons, Hawaiian wigglers, and the other fascinating lures would possibly stir a bit of the same excitement for my father that they did for me. I don't know why I never did it. Probably I feared that it would have no meaning for him and that I would open up the box and he would look inside, with curiosity perhaps, but mostly with perplexity and blankness. I guess I decided that this was a memory that belonged in the garage and should remain there.

* * *

During that month, and the next, I returned to the apartment to talk more with my mother. I wanted to be certain her decision hadn't changed. But every time I questioned her, she would cut me off.

"Don't keep talking about it," she would say. "I told you. I've made up my mind."

One night, after she had gone to sleep, I went out to the living room and spent some hours at my father's desk looking through more of the documents he'd left in its drawers when he had packaged up the larger body of materials and sent them to my home. In one of the folders that he hadn't labeled, I came across a copy of Eugene O'Neill's last will and testament, dated 1948, which Carlotta had apparently given to my father to keep in his office vault, for what reason I don't know (it would be rewritten twice before the playwright's death). I also found a number of letters from Carlotta to my father and, to my surprise, another last will and testament that O'Neill had written—this one for his dog!

I took the folder and some other items with me to my house so that I could look at them unhurriedly. The will and testament for the playwright's dog, a Dalmatian, Silverdene Emblem–"Blemie," as O'Neill had called him—was a lovely, sweet, and playful piece of writing that few people would have thought to be the product of a writer so bedeviled, grim, tumultuous, and deadly serious in his dark creative work.

"I, Silverdene Emblem O'Neill...," Blemie's

will began, "because the burden of my years and infirmities is heavy upon me, and I realize the end of my life is near, do hereby bury my last will and testament in the mind of my Master.... Now that I have grown blind and deaf and lame, and even my sense of smell fails me so that a rabbit could be right under my nose and I might not know..., I feel life is taunting me with having over-lingered.... It is time I said goodbye....

"Dogs do not fear death as men do. We accept it as a part of life.... What may come after death, who knows?" Blemie then suggested that if his master should decide to have another dog, he could not do better than to have another Dalmatian. "To him I bequeath my collar and leash and my overcoat and raincoat, made to order in 1929 at Hermès in Paris. He can never wear them with the distinction I did, walking around the Place Vendôme, or later along Park Avenue, all eyes fixed on me in admiration; but... I am sure he will do his utmost not to appear a mere gauche provincial dog."

In his "last word of farewell," Blemie left his master with the reassurance that, whenever he and his mistress came to visit at his grave, "no matter how deep my sleep I shall hear you, and not all the power of death can keep my spirit from wagging a grateful tail."

In the envelope containing Blemie's will there was a photograph of Blemie with O'Neill, the two of them resting on a sloping lawn, O'Neill leaning on one of his elbows, Blemie on his two front legs. It had been taken in 1931, when O'Neill was living on Long Island. "Mourning Becomes Electra was produced that fall in New York," Carlotta had noted on the back of the photograph in her flowing hand when she gave this to my father.

Even in the face of Carlotta's many acts of graciousness—she sent flowers to my mother now and then, usually with notes of extravagant affection—my father's annotations made it clear that he continued to regard her with a complicated mix of empathy, because of the injustice that was done to her when she was in McLean, and a painful sense of recognition that she could be unforgiving, "cruel and vengeful," in the way she treated others, even when she had good reason to dislike them. "Still hates Lawrence Langner of the Theatre Guild. Calls him 'son of a bitch,' because he called in Merrill to 'establish' her insanity...."

He noted that Carlotta could also be demeaning to O'Neill himself. More than once, when she was angry, she insulted him in my father's presence by disparaging his sexual performance, an insult that my father thought peculiarly gratuitous, and verging on the comical, in light of his medical debilitation. O'Neill, in turn, continually insulted her as well. When there was something he wanted her to do for him, he would yell out, "Where's my whore?" or, sometimes, "Goddamn whore?"

"You lousy bastard," she once answered. "Where

would you be today if it wasn't for this whore? In the gutter! Or in an insane asylum where your theater friends would probably have put you while they were busy peddling your plays!"

Even in the face of these unhappy altercations, my father noted once again that O'Neill depended on her for the very capable, if at times heavy-handed, way in which she managed his affairs. And, except for the times when he was most impatient or indignant with Carlotta, he never ceased to speak of her with gratitude for her unfailingly effective exercise of power when he was working in the fullness of his strength, because she used that power to defend him from distractions that might have intruded on the single-minded concentration that he needed "to release a work he had conceived" (those were my father's words) but which he felt at first was still entrapped within him.

In describing the protection that Carlotta had afforded him, he spoke about the sense of desperation he would feel as he grew immersed in the initial stages of creating a new play. He said he would experience "a gnawing sense of guilt at imprisoning what was in me and [was] struggling to come out. The only peace I ever had was made by myself by writing my plays."

At the same time, in spite of his reliance on Carlotta in helping him achieve the degree of isolation that he needed in these periods of writing, he also said that her determination to cut him off from all distractions, even those he might enjoy, remained undiminished even when he wasn't working on a play and, indeed, well into the years when he was unable to write any plays at all. He spoke, for instance, of the willfulness—"ferociousness," my father wrote— with which Carlotta fended off any mild interest other women now and then might show in him.

In one moment of revelatory reminiscence, O'Neill told my father of an actress named Patricia Neal, who, at the age of twenty, auditioned for a role in one of his plays. Although she didn't get the part, a pleasant friendship soon was formed between them. O'Neill confessed he found her "real attractive," "very pretty," and he said she brought him "flattery" and "adoration."

The relationship between the playwright and Ms. Neal, which had developed when his tremor was already quite pronounced and when he was hardly in a physical condition to carry on an amorous liaison with a twenty-year old girl, was, according to O'Neill, entirely innocent. He said he had "an ice cream soda" with her once and that their conversations had been casual and light-hearted, although he added that he kept these meetings secret from Carlotta and that, when she learned of them, she grew very angry.

"Hell! It wasn't worth it to me [i.e., to pursue the matter]. I needed Carlotta....She was my shield— and sometimes my captor."

Carlotta's uneasiness about O'Neill's friendship

with Patricia Neal remained unabated even after they had moved to Boston and O'Neill was in my father's care. In 1952, O'Neill confided to my father that he took much satisfaction at the news that the producer of a revival of one of his plays, Desire Under the Elms, was about to sign Patricia for a starring role. Carlotta, however, promptly intervened and ordered the producer to terminate negotiations.

Ms. Neal's career was later interrupted by a series of strokes that left her with a cerebral impairment, which she would struggle valiantly and, at length, successfully to overcome. She then returned to acting in a number of performances that brought her great acclaim. Carlotta's opposition to Patricia's wish to win a role for which O'Neill believed she was well suited was still in my father's mind and obviously rankled in his memory as late as 1968, when he saw a reference to Patricia in the New York Times.

"Brave woman....Did I ever tell you that O'Neill was rather fond of her?"

Carlotta's domination of O'Neill's decision making extended even into areas in which my father found that he himself was innocently involved. O'Neill, for instance, mentioned to him once that he liked to listen to the ball games on the radio. My father quickly seized on this and asked O'Neill if he'd like to go with him to see a game at Fenway Park, which was just a couple blocks from O'Neill's hotel.

O'Neill "reacted like a kid," my father noted–

"almost boyishly enthusiastic"—"but Carlotta vetoed…." In a query to himself, he wondered what she possibly could have objected to. Did she think the two of them would disappear, "make a jailbreak," and decide not to return? Even with her total faith in my father's judgment in matters that had any real significance, the notion of her husband and his doctor going off to have an afternoon together at the ballpark seemed to pose a threat to her.

On a far more serious note, she forcefully resisted any inclinations O'Neill would now and then express to get in touch with his daughter, Oona, from whom he'd been distanced since she was a girl of seventeen because he had disapproved of the lively social life she led, which was highly publicized in newspaper columns and which he believed to be an exploitation of his name and reputation. His disapproval grew considerably greater only a year later when she fell in love with a much older man, the actor Charlie Chaplin, and in short order married him.

O'Neill had since had second thoughts about his harshness to his daughter, but Carlotta remained adamant in her hostility to Oona. When, in 1953, the Boston Globe published a photo of Oona and her children, my father wrote, "Showed it to EO'N, but had to do it surreptitiously. Carlotta noted same in paper, crumpled it, and canceled [their] subscription."

Some years after "EO'N" had passed away,

Oona had written to my father from her home in Switzerland. "Very hurt…, [she] confided later," according to one of the memos filed in another folder that contained his correspondence with her. Having been excluded from her father's life for more than a decade when he died, Oona now experienced a yearning to know more about him and his state of mind, his regrets or recollections, in the years in which my father treated him. She asked my father if he would agree to visit her in Switzerland.

He wasn't sure at first if it was wise for him to do this. The relationship between the playwright and his daughter had been disrupted for so long, and under conditions that had been so difficult for Oona, that my father worried that a lengthy conversation might simply open up old wounds and would not assuage her longings but, instead, might deepen them. On the other hand, there were statements that O'Neill had made in reference to his daughter, and out of the hearing of Carlotta, that conveyed a tenderness of which my father was convinced that Oona could not be aware. In one moment of reflection, for example, he had spoken lovingly of Oona when she was a child, and he remembered with remorse the way he had reacted to the independent choices she was making in her teenage years.

"She—*tiny* she—gave me strength [and] seemed to be hovering over me like an angel. Hell! I was afraid of her and yet I loved this tiny mite. God-damned selfish of me," he had said, "oblivious to [the] harm I did to her.... When she kicked up her heels in a restaurant with her society friends, I scolded her [in] a letter. What in hell right did I have to do this? I had abandoned them"—a reference to both Oona and her brother, Shane—"and their mother," who was a writer by the name of Agnes Boulton, to whom O'Neill was married at the time he met Carlotta.

After having made this reference to abandonment, O'Neill had asked my father, "Do you know what it is to have a guilty conscience?" Then, before my father could reply: "Is there any other kind?"

In speaking of Chaplin, O'Neill had told my father, "When she married him, I blamed myself. I took it as self-retribution," but, he added, "he will do better by her than I." In a bracketed passage, my father noted that O'Neill's use of the future tense ("he will do better") gave the impression that he still was thinking of her as the teenage daughter she had been at the time she married.

"Harry," he said, "take care of her. She deserves it more than I." My father had written, again in brackets, "This perplexed me." But, because he didn't demur at this request, he believed that he had made a kind of promise.

The only other item in this file, a memo written on a piece of stationery from a grand hotel in Switzerland—the letterhead reads "Le Beau Rivage"—reminded me that my father had finally accepted Oona's invitation and had traveled to Switzerland with my mother and talked with Oona and her husband at their home in a village called Corsier-sur-Vevey, about a dozen miles from Lausanne. "I felt obliged to keep my promise…, and I did. Oona cried softly," my father wrote, apparently on the evening after they had had this conversation—the first of several, it would seem.

Reading these materials, written by my father so many years before, I was reminded once again of the depth of loyalty he'd felt to a man regarded often as a cold and distant person who was loyal, for his own part, only to his creativity. The rapidly developing intensity of my father's attachment to O'Neill—or "Gene," as he would call him in the course of conversations—had led into the most consuming and exacting medical relationship of his career. But the satisfaction he derived from giving up the better part of two and a half years to the service of an author he revered was, I knew, beyond all measure to my father.

O'Neill, in his belief—and in the belief, I think, of most historians of theater—was not merely one more gifted author of distinguished works of drama along with maybe half a dozen other major playwrights that our nation had produced. In the grandeur of his reach, in the power of his capability to make us rage and weep, he belonged, as most critics saw it, in the company of August Strindberg, Henrik Ibsen, and the great French classicists Corneille and Racine—and "at least in some proximity," as my father ventured once, "to the Greek tragedians…."

Suddenly now to have the opportunity to know this man in his emotional completeness and to try, with all the skill at his command, to ease the turmoil that O'Neill had suffered for so long was, for my father, a culminating moment in his clinical experience. This is why I've felt the obligation to pass on what he entrusted to me in its near entirety, even in its passages of unimportant acrimony or literary marginality, and even in some instances of playful triviality.

Once, by way of playfulness, O'Neill took off his bathrobe—an expensive one, my father said, that Carlotta probably had bought him in one of the boutique shops she frequented in Paris or New York—and insisted that my father put it on during an examination. "It gives you the appearance of being quite distinguished," he observed. My father said he knew that he was being teased, because O'Neill was rather tall "and the robe was much too big for me." O'Neill, he said, "laughed outrageously to see me standing there, trying to be serious, in a robe that nearly reached the floor."

Summer was nearly over now, and my dog Persnickety, who had brought so much delight and love into my father's life, was suffering from a rapid growth in her malignancy. Up until the recent months, the cancer had progressed more slowly than the doctor had expected, but the period of grace Persnickety had been allowed was coming to an end. By the last week of August, her right eye was completely closed. She no longer had the strength to come upstairs and sleep beside me, and she had begun to lose her appetite and would eat only if I fed her with my hand. I knew the time would soon arrive when it would be wrong for me to try to keep her in this world.

One night, I put her in my car and brought her with me for a final visit with my father. She was too weak to climb up on his knees or play the games of throw-and-fetch my father had enjoyed. She curled up on the rug in front of him and, when he reached down to stroke her ears, she licked his fingers and looked up at him. That was about the most that she could manage now.

The owners of the building in which my mother lived had changed their animal-friendly policy a year before. So my mother hadn't seen Persnickety except on one occasion in the winter, eight months earlier, when I was able to convince the woman who signed in people at the door to break the rules and let Persnickety come upstairs with me in order to surprise my mother on her birthday.

At that time, Persnickety was not too lethargic to race into my mother's room the way she'd always done, hop up on my mother's bed, and slobber her with kisses on her mouth and forehead. My mother didn't object at all to letting Persnickety sit there, virtually on top of her. Then Persnickety ran into the living room, found a bear my mother had given her, which had been propped up on a chair, took it in her teeth, brought it to the far end of the room, and shook it back and forth relentlessly.

A week later, my mother said she'd had a dream about Persnickety. "We had taken her to the Four Seasons"—she and my father sometimes went for dinner there before he became ill—"and there was a group of little girls who were playing in the lobby. She was wearing a wide pink ribbon which the girls had placed around her neck and they made a circle around her and they danced and sang a song, 'The Farmer in the Dell,' and she began to dance with them!

"She danced so nicely on her little feet that everybody was amazed." A man in the lobby who, my mother said, "was in the movie business," went to a phone and called a movie agent "and they decided to make a movie of Persnickety dancing right there in the lobby!"

On another night, she had another dream about Persnickety. A boy I'd known when I was a teenager, before I went to college, whom she had never liked, had tried to kill Persnickety. In her dream, my father had said, "I never trusted him, and I was right. I always knew he had a twisted personality." But she also said that, in her dream, she had asked herself, "Is this really happening? Am I awake? Or am I only dreaming?"

In subsequent months, she questioned me about Persnickety. She knew I'd managed once to get her into the apartment since the rules were changed, so she grew suspicious as to why I didn't bring her there again. As the summer went on and the tumor grew much larger, I tried to give my mother nonspecific answers. But her investigative instincts proved to be too sharp for me to fool her very long. Under her interrogation, I at last told her the truth.

"I knew it," she said, not as kindly as I would have liked, because she knew I'd been deceiving her.

On August 25, she said she had this dream: "You sleep upstairs and there is a narrow stairway and sometimes Persnickety gets up from the bed and goes down to the living room. You woke up one night and you saw she wasn't there, so you went downstairs and found her on the sofa. You sat with her and held her in your arms and she looked up at you, but her eyes were very sad and she wasn't moving...."

By the time my mother had that dream, Persnickety was no longer strong enough to go out into the garden. I put newspapers near the kitchen door and she reverted to the habit she had had when she was a puppy and I had been training her. The day arrived, soon after that, when she would no longer eat at all, even when I tempted her with her favorite treats. I called the veterinarian who had taken care of her since she'd been a few weeks old. He was kind enough to offer to drive over to my house to put Persnickety to sleep.

After I had buried her in the garden where she used to play, I drove into Boston to be with my mother. I never got to finish the first sentence I began. As soon as I spoke Persnickety's name, she lifted her arthritic hand and placed it on my arm. Julia was sitting with us in the bedroom. She later observed that my mother, fragile and dependent and distracted by her fantasies as she often was, had not lost the fortitude to connect directly with a painful moment of reality.

"This is the penalty we pay," my mother said.

"Penalty, Mrs. Kozol?" Julia asked.

"The penalty for love," my mother quietly replied.

Julia went into the kitchen then. When the tea was ready, we helped my mother walk into the dining room.

Julia had a skillful way of settling my mother down into her chair. After we had had our tea, my mother asked if I would go and find the picture I had taken of Persnickety when she was a puppy, which was on the bureau in the bedroom. Once I placed the picture in her hands, she said that she would like to stay there in the dining room a while.

"You can go now," she instructed me.

Julia went out in the corridor with me. I think she knew I would have liked to stay there with my mother for a little longer. The sudden sense of emptiness awaiting me at home was going to be hard for me.

It was mid-September now. I had delayed for the entire summer in putting aside my final hesitations about Daddy. In the ultimate event, it was not my mother's firm determination, or the reinforcement I was being given by the other people I had turned to for advice, but an unexpected piece of information I was given by my father's trust attorney, that impelled me to move forward.

I had asked him several times over the preceding years if the funds he was investing for my parents would be enough to meet the very high expense of paying for the nursing home (the portion of that cost not covered by insurance or by Medicare), the extra attendants that were needed by my father, those that were needed by my mother, as well as my mother's rent and food and all the other costs for the apartment. He had routinely answered that there was no reason for concern. "Your mother and father are in good financial shape," or words to that effect. As recently as three years before, he had pegged their assets at about $2 million.

Suddenly now, and only when I asked him, he told me that their total wealth, which had lost one quarter of its value in the market downturn that year and the two preceding years, would be depleted, at the present rate of their expenditures, in approximately eighteen months.

At a meeting in which we did some hasty mathematics, he concluded that, with the subtraction of the nursing home expenses and a few additional adjustments, some of which might call for my ability to underwrite a portion of the salaries for those who would take care of them at home, my parents' assets would not likely be exhausted for as long as three more years. At that time, if my mother and father—or either one of them—were still alive, they would be penniless.

The next day I sat down with Silvia and asked if it was possible for her to extricate herself from any obligations she was under to the agency for which she had been working, in order to save the large amount of money the company was charging for its services. She told me that she didn't think this would be a problem. (The agency director, once she understood the situation, gave us her agreement.) Silvia also said she'd want to have another talk with Julia so that they could figure out how many extra people they would need, especially when either she or Julia had to be away.

I had joked with Silvia sometimes in the past about her strong "take-over" inclinations. Now I found myself indebted to her for those qualities. She moved into action with a furious determination to arrange things in a manner that would leave me free to act upon the many other details I would have to handle quickly.

Lucinda, when I told her I had come to a decision, agreed to oversee the physical condition of my father on at least an intermittent basis in between her other obligations. Although she was prepared to do this without payment, I persuaded her to let me pay a modest sum, since she had a family to support and also had tuition costs to meet, because she had begun a course of training to become a nurse practitioner.

It was Silvia and Julia, however, whom I would inevitably rely upon the most. Without them, I could not have brought my father home. Although a schedule was arranged in which the hours of two helpers would overlap for long enough that they could assist each other with some portions of the work that were impossible to do alone, there would also be long stretches of each day when one of them would find herself entirely on her own.

The responsibility these women would sustain was going to require an unusual degree of moral stamina. In the absence of the close attention I had hoped for but in fact could not always count on from the geriatric specialist in Boston who would soon take on the role of primary physician for my father, Silvia and Julia would become the only thoroughly reliable and rapidly reactive health providers for the last years of his life.

Those who work as home attendants and companions to the elderly are given little of the respect and, of course, a great deal less of the remuneration that are given to physicians and others in the higher reaches of the healthcare industry. But in many situations they are the only ones who truly *know* the patients and the ones who advocate with greatest diligence on their behalf. My father had always liked the word "clinician" better than "physician" because it held the connotation of direct, unmediated, never arm's-length service to the people he'd been asked to care for. In this respect, it was the ever-loyal and perpetually watchful Julia and Silvia who came to be my father's actual clinicians—all the more so as they gained in expertise by questioning Lucinda and by watching carefully when, as his condition might require, visiting nurses were dispatched to the apartment to examine him.

All this was still ahead of us, however. Once I had convinced myself that Silvia and Julia had things under good control, I gave official notice to the nursing home. My father would be leaving on October 10.

"Are we going home?" he asked after I had spent a final evening with him at the nursing home, as he'd asked with various degrees of urgency or wistfulness so many times before.

"Yes, Daddy," I replied. "This time, we really are."

CHAPTER EIGHT

A Sense of Exploration

Silvia and Julia had made careful preparations. A wheelchair had been rented, and a hospital bed and various instruments to check my father's vital signs had been set up in the smaller bedroom, directly adjacent to the room in which my mother slept.

My mother went to sleep much later than my father. Her first question when she awoke was: "Did you wake the baby?" Then she would ask, "Did you give him his breakfast? Did you cook his oatmeal for him?" She had told Silvia: "He likes his oatmeal with a little cream and just a bit of sugar."

After he had breakfast, Silvia or Julia would bring him to the living room. Later in the morning, my mother would come out to keep him company. They would often have their lunch together in the

dining area. Then my mother went back to her bedroom, while my father would remain there in the
living room, usually sitting at his desk, as he'd done
before he became ill.

The surface of the desk and a table to its side
continued to be piled up with newly arriving medical journals, as well as bulletins and correspondence
from neurological and psychiatric institutes and
occasional letters, from the dean of Harvard Medical
School for instance, offering him congratulations on
his birthdays or maybe simply making an announce-
ment about upcoming seminars or conferences to
which alumni were invited.

Julia also told me he was still receiving letters
from people who had no idea how old he was or that
he was ill, asking his opinion of an academic paper
or, perhaps, soliciting his observations on a research
study being carried out in one of those areas in which
he had specialized. Since she knew he couldn't read
and understand these letters, she would often read
them to him. If she held a letter right in front of him,
she said, "he would look at it over and over" and
would sometimes point to something that appeared
to hold a glint of meaning to him, and she said he'd
nod at times, as if in recognition of a name or institution, and might make a brief remark to indicate his
satisfaction.

He also began again to make brief jottings to
himself—words or phrases, chaotic in their form and
with no apparent continuity. He used the same blue

sheets of fine-grained paper he had used in writing memos to himself for much of his career, which were in a wooden tray on the right front corner of his desk, where they had always been.

Now and then he'd look into the desk and come upon an object that attracted his attention. One day, for example, he took out the nameplate, made of heavy metal, with the letters of his name corroded slightly, tinged in green, that had once adorned his office door. "He lingered over it," said Julia. "He just kept on looking at it for the longest time…." He'd also sometimes pull out file cards, look at them, one after another, then when he was finished he would try to put them back where they belonged.

I didn't think my father's interest in these items, or the random and staccato jottings that he made, were indications of a sudden restoration of some long-departed portion of his memory. I certainly did not believe that he was thinking to himself, "This is my office. This is the desk at which I used to work." But Julia said she was convinced that he felt "some kind of connection" to that desk because he had a proud and confident expression when he sat there.

One of the items he took out of the desk was a stiff manila envelope that was filled with photographs he'd taken, and addresses he had written, some of them in German. On the front of the envelope there was a notation: "Follow up—Vienna."

Julia showed the pictures to my mother, who told her they were from a trip they made, sometime in the 1950s, for a meeting with a group of Eastern European doctors who had managed somehow to obtain permission to travel to Vienna to confer with Western European and American physicians. Julia said that she became quite animated when she spoke of what she called "a secret meeting" in a room at their hotel with "a brilliant woman, a Hungarian psychiatrist," who was planning to escape from Budapest and was looking for my father's help in finding a position at one of the psychiatric centers in New York or Boston.

Julia said my mother also told her they had traveled to Vienna on a famous train known as the Orient Express, which "began in Paris and went all the way to Istanbul," or she may have said "Constantinople." She said they had their own compartment but a young romantic couple they encountered in the dining car were so enjoyable to be with that they stayed up very late to talk with them and then met them in the morning to have breakfast.

Julia left the envelope on my father's desk so I could see the pictures. There were several of my mother standing on a sidewalk in front of the State Opera in Vienna. The others were apparently of doctors they had met. Then I returned it to the drawer where she said he'd found it. None of this, said Julia, seemed to have much meaning for my father.

Of all the items he had taken from his desk, only the corroded nameplate from his former office door seemed to have stirred up some truly strong emotion. "It *did* mean something to him," Julia said. "You could tell. The way he traced the outline of the letters with his fingers....I don't know"—her voice choked up—"it made me feel like crying."

In that first year after he came home, he would often have his dinner at the dining table or while sitting at his desk. Silvia said she knew he liked the meals she cooked, because he ate voraciously. She also noted other aspects of his physical vitality, including the persistence of his sexual awareness and self-consciousness. "When I bathe him," she reported, "he becomes embarrassed by his naked-ness. But he sometimes reaches out and tries to touch my bosom. And when I turn around to get a towel, he reaches up and grabs me by the bottom!"

One afternoon, Silvia said, her husband came to meet my father and remained to visit for a while. "Your father was very polite to him at first," she said. He looked her husband up and down and seemed to have decided he approved of him.

"Sir," he said, "I think you are a gentleman."

I don't know exactly what my father did at that point. He may have reached for Silvia's arm or put his hand around her waist. Whatever it was, Silvia's husband took it in good humor and did his best to make a joke out of the situation. "Hey, watch it! That's my wife!" he said with pretended sternness.

But Silvia said that Daddy did not find this to his liking. "He's not a gentleman after all," he said and turned away from him.

"As soon as my husband left the room, your father brightened up. He had me to himself again, which is the way he liked it."

Did he enjoy the fact that he was home? The answer, Silvia believed, was obvious. Once, when he had to spend a few days at the hospital and "the ambulance man," as Silvia said, brought him home and came upstairs and helped to put him back in bed, my father began to clap his hands. "He was *clapping*!" she repeated.

I asked her if she meant that he was doing this to thank the man for helping him. "No," she said. "Not for the ambulance man. It was for himself! It was like, 'I'm home again!' It was a celebration!"

My mother was happy he was home, but naturally, with her state of mind so clear, my father couldn't offer her the company or conversation she enjoyed. After he had gone to sleep, Silvia or Julia would have dinner with her. Then they would sit up with her to watch the ball games or the news, or simply chat with her until her eyes began to close.

"Once," Silvia told me, "when your mother closed her eyes and I thought she was asleep, I switched the channel to the Spanish-language station. She suddenly sat up, wide awake, and she seemed confused. She told me, 'I don't understand a word they're speaking.' It's a noisy program. She thought there was something wrong with her because she couldn't understand the voices. Then she looked more closely at the screen and I could see she was relieved. She'd figured it out. She said, 'I know. I understand what I don't understand. It's because it's Spanish.' "

Before she fell asleep that night, she asked if Silvia would "go in and check the baby." Her solicitude on his behalf was only intermittent at the start, but after a few months went by she seemed to grow more tender and protective.

In the second year after my father had come home, he developed an infection in his urinary tract, which had been a problem a couple times before while he was in the nursing home. When it recurred and then worsened rapidly in December of that year, Julia tried to reach his doctor, but, when she had no success, she telephoned Lucinda and, at her advice, she called an ambulance and brought him to the hospital.

When they got there, Julia said, the woman at the registration desk wasn't very friendly. "She didn't want to let him in. I had his Medicare card and his insurance information, but she wouldn't look at them. That's the only time that's ever happened there. I don't know what her problem was. I had to plead with her.

" 'Why did you bring him here?' she asked.

" 'Because he's sick,' I said.

" 'How do you know?' the woman said. 'He can't even talk.'

"I was so angry! He was right in front of her. 'Babies cannot talk,' I told her, 'but we know when they're in pain.'"

The woman at last reluctantly admitted him. He was seen by a physician who confirmed that Julia's judgment was correct.

He remained in the hospital for three or four days. After the infection was brought under control, the doctor taking care of him told me that, in view of his history of similar infections and the severity of this one, it would be advisable to have his urine tested weekly after his release. He said that this should be a standing policy from this time on, with antibiotics prescribed without delay if indications of infection were to reappear.

Julia had left a message for his doctor when she took my father to the hospital, but neither of us knew how long it was before she got the message and went in to visit him. Julia said she thought the doctor had been out of town, so it's possible she didn't get to see him in the hospital.

Once he was home, I sent her a fax about the weekly urine testing recommended at the hospital. She replied that this was acceptable to her. I told her that Lucinda would be glad to take the samples. She answered that this plan was "satisfactory."

I was troubled, however, that this plan of action had not been proposed by her but had to be suggested by another doctor. I was also perplexed that, knowing of my father's history, she had not initiated any plan like this prior to the time when an advanced infection had required him to be admitted to the hospital.

It was another year and a half before my father had to be admitted to the hospital again. In this case, the antibiotic he'd been taking when it had been needed to suppress infection in his urinary tract had ceased to be effective. Again, his own physician could not be reached for several days. Her office said she was away.

It was a resident at the MGH who told me the infection had, among its consequences, led to a fluttering of my father's heart. ("Atrial fibrillation" was the term he used and then defined for me in words that I could understand.) Once he was stabilized, the doctor said a new and stronger antibiotic ought to be prescribed to counter the resistant organism that had led to a recurrence of infection.

The day before my father was sent home, his geriatrician told me that, since she had returned, she had given information on his status to Lucinda, even though Lucinda had been at the hospital and had been following the situation closely while the doctor was away. The doctor said she had decided to prescribe a stronger medication.

I need to pause here to explain the feelings that were running through my mind about the geriatric specialist who'd been recommended to me for my father's care. First of all, it is only accurate to note that, as a member of one of the medical groups in the Boston area, she was always able to rely upon the services of one of her associates when she was out of town. And, when my father was sick enough to be admitted to the hospital, I knew that he would not be left without the treatment he required.

What I found more than a little maddening, however, and Silvia and Julia considerably more so, was the lack of continuity in dealing with his doctor and the difficulty that we faced in getting through to her directly, and without inordinate delay. By way of contrast, my mother's physician, who was one of the busiest and most sought-after doctors in the city, was almost always rapidly available. When Silvia thought my mother ought to be examined, for whatever reason—she was having problems with her legs, for instance, which at times became severely swollen—I would call her doctor or, more commonly, Silvia would call him on her own, and, if he was busy when she called, she said he always called her back before he left his office for the day.

It was, she said, entirely different with my father's doctor. "Some other person in the office is the one I have to deal with...." Even when the doctor did return a call, she sometimes seemed dismissive of Silvia's concerns. When Silvia requested a flu shot for my father, for example, at the onset of cold weather, the doctor told her she didn't think that this was really needed, and, besides, she said she didn't have "supplies available." Silvia, whose children and grandchildren had just had their flu shots, was unwilling to accept this. Instead of wasting time in pestering the doctor, she called my mother's primary physician.

"It's essential," he advised her. "Bring him in the first thing in the morning before my office opens." I regretted that he was unable to take on my father as his full-time patient. But the point that counted at the moment was that Silvia had the common sense and activist mentality not to let the geriatric doctor deny my father something that he needed, and at the time he needed it.

There was another, and more complicated, issue that I needed to confront in my dealings with his doctor. For reasons I will clarify in greater detail later on, I had refused to sign a document known as a DNR—"Do Not Resuscitate"—which is commonly agreed to by the healthcare proxy in the case of someone of my father's age and physical and cerebral condition. Instead, I had insisted that my father be on "full code" when he was in the hospital, a policy his doctor seemed to have accepted once I reinforced it to her personally but which she told me was regarded as "unusual" for someone in his situation. What troubled me was not that medical professionals working with the elderly might find my wish, as she had said, unusual or even inappropriate. The problem, for me, was the formulaic way in which the larger question underlying all of this was almost automatically addressed.

What I mean is that his doctor and, on occasion,

others who were tending to my father, when they spoke to me about his situation, tended to employ what always sounded like a scripted nostrum, redolent of what one might expect to find in books of pop psychology, about "the quality of life" versus the worth of life itself. There was also something in the way they spoke that led me to believe that they perceived themselves as ethicists—specialists, as it were, in the theology of life and death—a perception to which I felt they had no rightful claim. In some instances, moreover, I was given the uneasy feeling that the high-minded ethical positions they assumed on the point at which a person's life no longer ought to be preserved might be an unconscious or only semiconscious way to reconcile professional integrity with the economics of the healthcare system and with that larger set of economic values that increasingly determine medical priorities in the United States.

In any event, so long as my father still took even modest amounts of satisfaction in his daily life—and I relied far more on Silvia's and Julia's and my own perceptions on this matter than those of physicians who might spend no more than thirty minutes in his presence at a time—I thought his doctor ought to be as diligent in coming up with good preventive and protective measures for my father, and without my being forced to beg for them, as pediatricians, for example, normally would do in treatment of a child who might suffer from a neurological impairment.

In this respect, I could never quite get over

the debilitating sense that I was pulling constantly against a very heavy weight, not of outright opposition on the doctor's part, but of passivity, procrastination, and inertia. "If you suggest it, and insist upon it, then I will agree to do it." That's essentially the message that I got. But, even after we had come to an agreement on one area of treatment, the problem would come up again in a different context.

At the same time, and making things a good deal more complex for me, I could never totally suppress the recognition, or at least suspicion, that much of my irritation with my father's doctor served as a distraction for me from a wholly different matter that I knew had no direct connection with his actual well-being. At some level, I think I was aware that selfish motivations of my own might very likely be at stake in the decisions I was making. As I imagine many people who have been in my position will not find it hard to understand, the truth is that I did not want to let my father die because I could not picture life within this world without him. As nonresponsive as he often was, and physically enfeebled as he had become, I could not escape the crazy thought that I still needed him.

A sensitive young doctor, a resident in cardiology who attended to my father once when he was in the hospital, spoke with me of my concerns and, although we didn't have much time to talk, she said she'd keep in touch with me. She later wrote me a reflective letter in which she, who was the daughter and granddaughter of physicians, told me that she was at home and dealing with the same dilemma, in the case of her grandmother, that she and I had talked about when we were standing at the nurses' station just a few feet from my father's door.

"We are facing the same decision you are facing with your father. It is so unbelievably striking for me to be on the other side of this decision-making process—unbelievable, I mean, that, in this family of so many doctors, we are unable to make decisions about my grandmother's care, because so many of us are unready to let go. It is so hard to tease out what we are holding onto for our own sakes, as opposed to hers.

"That said, I am enjoying my time with her so much. She is the most brilliant woman I have ever met. She is totally demented now, and has been for some time, but her delusions are so consistent!" (This part made me think about my mother, who, though certainly not "demented," did, as we have seen, indulge her fantasies—delusions, if that is the proper word—which were consistent too.)

Her grandmother's delusions, she went on, had to do with ordinary details of caring for her family—"getting me married," "fixing my hair...." Before departing for the hospital, she said, her grandmother had been "sitting on her bed, phone in hand, trying to reschedule a hair appointment. This was her fixation....

"I know you are going through similar things. I just understand now more than ever."

When we had a chance to meet again and share our feelings on these matters at much greater length, I asked her if she'd thought at all about the question of priorities to which I have referred in drawing a comparison between what I had seen of geriatric care and what I knew of other fields of medicine, including pediatrics. I told her I believed that what I'd been observing seemed to offer evidence of something that may well appear, from a purely economic point of view, to be an absolutely rational distinction in the valuation of the worth of human life. A child—or anyone who's relatively young—has, potentially at least, a life of productivity ahead. A ninety-eight-year-old neurologist who suffers from dementia has no further value to the economic order.

I told her I could not help thinking that the willingness to relegate a person in my father's situation to a lower and less vigilant degree of medical attention was an accurate reflection of the values of a social system which, as I had learned in my own work in education, measures human life, more frequently than not, in rather hard-nosed and explicit terms of future payoff to the national well-being. ("Future productivity" is one of the most commonly heard phrases used in governmental circles to justify expenditures for preschool or for early infant care. "These babies, if well treated now, will someday be taxpayers and contribute to our national prosperity." Elderly and unwell people will, of course, contribute nothing to our national prosperity. They are simply "sitting there," using up the wealth of those who still pay taxes.)

As a physician who had come to her vocation with the highest possible ideals of selflessness and service, she was not prepared to countenance the likelihood that economic valuations of a patient's "worth to the society" would ever be permitted to intrude upon the life-preserving obligations of a member of the medical profession. She did, however, recognize, although somewhat reluctantly, that structural arrangements, or financial limitations, or governmentally established policy decisions, might have the effect of making it more difficult for doctors to fulfill these obligations.

She also noted that the field of geriatrics has not been accorded the level of prestige that many other areas of medicine command and that the pay scale is far less than in most other specialties. As a consequence, she said, not enough doctors of her age, burdened by the heavy loans they've incurred to pay for their tuition, were being drawn into this specialty. The number of geriatricians, accordingly, was insufficient to address the needs of the increasingly large numbers of the elderly, and those who did sustain positions in this field had much larger caseloads than would be the norm in other areas of care. This, she said, might help explain the difficulties Silvia and I encountered with my father's doctor.

An older physician whom I also questioned told me that he thought her speculations were correct, although he urged me not to paint the situation with too broad a brush, because he said that people drawn to geriatrics tended to be motivated by profound compassion. "They tend to be unselfish people. Many come into this field after they've been through the same things you've been facing, with *their* parents or grandparents." Then, too, he made the point that the doctor caring for my father might well have academic or collegial obligations competing for her time and that this might be one reason she was out of town or unavailable so frequently.

If that was the case, I asked, wouldn't it have been appropriate for her to have explained this to me from the start and perhaps referred me to another doctor who was less distracted by competing obligations?

"Ah," he replied, "but nobody, no physician, wants it to be thought that, amidst their other obligations, they cannot deliver on the needs of their own patients. That would be a terribly embarrassing concession. And I'm speaking now of *any* area of medicine...."

Having said this much, he told me that he didn't see that I had any choice but to be as stubborn and persistent as I had the will to be in pressing for the kind of care I thought my father needed and deserved. For this and other reasons, I do not regret one bit that I pressured and pursued my father's doctor as I did. If anything, I wish that I had done it more relentlessly.

There is a final point I ought to make about the sheer intensity and persistence of the bond that held me to my father. Although I know this may seem hard to understand, I think that I felt even closer to him now than I had been *before* the early indications of his illness. As I have mentioned, there had been extended periods when I had allowed the pressures of my work to distance me from both my parents and when I had seen them only at infrequent intervals. But since my father had grown ill, I had set aside entire weeks, and sometimes months, to be with him as often as I could and had probably spent more hours with him than I'd done at any time since I was a boy. I'd been listening with more attentiveness to almost every word he spoke, noticing his shifting moods and altering expressions, his evanescent bursts of gaiety, his times of relaxation and serenity when we were sitting, for example, on the patio outside of the nursing home and my dog was lying at his feet.

I have said I felt that I was on a journey with my father. Our guessing games while he was in the nursing home to try to fathom something that he wanted to express but could not lucidly convey, were one part of that journey. So, too, were our shared attempts to extricate a memory or penetrate a bafflement or navigate an interesting maze of interrupted reasoning. In these ways, I felt that we were joined to one another in an exploration not just of his own impeded processes of thought but of the mystery of thinking in itself. In this sense of exploration, I felt a more direct and intimate connection with my father than at almost any time since we went out on those evening walks together more than sixty years before when he was feeling discontent about his work, as my mother had explained, and seemed to get some comfort from my company.

If I hadn't spent so many hours with him in the nursing home but had managed to distract myself more thoroughly from his predicament by opportunities afforded by my work and by my friendships and political activities, and had made only limited and periodic visits, it would have been easier to look upon him now with a degree of distance, and through a lens of pathos, as if he were no longer the father I had known, but only a diminished version of that man. But I had made my choice and, as a consequence, I did not see him in that way at all.

Yes, it is true I'd been deeply shaken as I had observed the progress of an illness that had robbed my father of the gifts of clarity and insight that had made him a remarkable physician. But those gifts, those areas of competence, had never been the whole of who he was. In terms of his inherent charm and sweetness, and his humor, and his outright sense of mischief when he flirted with Lucinda or tried to get his hands on Silvia's rear end, but, most of all, in his long and brave and dignified resistance to the darkness that progressively encircled him, there was, for me, no diminution—not in the essence of the person he had been, not in the admiration that I felt for him. This is why it was so hard to let him go. The young doctor understood this.

CHAPTER NINE

My Father and Mother: Together and Apart

For the remainder of my parents' lives, Silvia or Julia was with them almost every day and every night. The exceptions were on weekends or, very rarely, on a weekday when both of them had to be away. At those times, one or another of the extra helpers Silvia had found would come in and take their place.

One of the best of these extra helpers was the wife of Alejandro, who, like Alejandro, had studied medicine in Cuba. (He had been a cardiologist; she had specialized in family medicine.) Sometimes Alejandro would come with her and stay there for an afternoon, helping when she needed help but mostly simply spending time in Daddy's company. Lucinda had, by now, become a nurse practitioner and no longer had the time to visit the apartment on a routine basis, so I was grateful for Alejandro's efforts to look for ways to make connections with my father and stir up his alertness.

Throughout his first two years at home, my father seemed to recognize me when I came into the room so long as I arrived before he had grown sleepy. When I kissed him, he would kiss me back. If he found it difficult to summon up my name, I would lean forward and whisper in his ear, "Hi, Daddy! It's me! It's Jonathan." He would smile and grasp my hand and look at me with that penetrating gaze that, no matter how impaired his memory might be, always seemed to indicate discernment.

Although his ability to carry on a conversation of any length at all had pretty much disappeared at least a year before, he surprised me now and then by the bluntness of an answer he would give to something I had asked. Once, after the second time he'd been in the hospital, a medication he'd been given led to a week of miserable diarrhea. When I asked how he was feeling—it was a dumb question—he gave me an awful look and answered, "Ich bin dreck"—meaning, more or less, "I feel like shit."

When he was alone with Julia and Silvia, the words he spoke were often in reaction to an act of kindness on their part or, in the case of Silvia, to something she had done that had aroused his anger. Once, when she was bathing him, she said that his resistance to her washing of his "private parts" (that, or "privates," was the term that she and Julia always used), with which she was familiar now, impelled him suddenly to challenge her with heated indignation.

"You're not going to get it!" he announced to her.

"I said to him, 'I don't *want* it, Dr. Kozol! I don't need it! I have a husband of my own.'"

I asked her if this made him laugh.

"No," she said. "He didn't laugh. He looked as if I'd startled him. I think he was a little shocked that I would say something like that."

My father's sense of sexual self-consciousness continued to be obvious to Silvia and Julia for a long time after he came home. When a visiting nurse arrived once every month to put in a new catheter— he had become incontinent by now—he would try to block her hands. "He'd cross his hands over his lap," Julia said, "as soon as she approached him and removed his covers. His arms were strong. He'd lock his hands together."

Then, once Julia had persuaded him to let the woman do her job, "he'd turn his head away from her and look at me with terrible embarrassment, as if he was thinking, 'Here's this woman who's a stranger to me and she's holding my privates in her hand.' It was like, 'What's this woman trying to do to me?' He was relieved the moment she was gone."

My father was sleeping longer now, falling asleep about an hour earlier than when he first came home, but Julia and Silvia made it a point to keep him up most of the day. They would lift him from his wheelchair and would lead him back and forth in the apartment or outside in the hallway, as they still did with my mother, to make him exercise his legs and keep his circulation strong.

When he was sitting at his desk, said Julia, he continued "to try to write things to himself"—letters and numbers, fragments of words, sometimes an entire word, with arrows often pointing from one word or letter to another. "It was like doodling," she said, but the letters and numbers, as before, were recognizable. At times, she noticed, there would be an element of urgency or even mild franticness in the way he did this, putting aside one piece of paper, then reaching for another.

In the evenings I would see those papers scattered on his desk. The arrows and lines connecting words or numbers, frequently darting up and down a page between two separate items, gave the impression of that sense of hecticness and urgency that Julia had described. It was as if he were racing the clock, getting down these messages, or meanings, or reminders to himself while he still had the chance. Julia said that he looked "very busy" while he did these writings.

Late at night, once my mother was asleep, I would sometimes sit there at my father's desk and take out some envelopes and folders from one of the drawers, as I'd done when he was in the nursing home. A number of folders, buried beneath other items—long-outdated legal documents, insurance applications, greeting cards, drafts of letters he may or may not have mailed—opened up entire chapters in his life that I hadn't thought about for years. As with the items on O'Neill, I brought these folders to my house and stayed up for several nights recapturing some of the most intriguing moments of transition in his medical career.

One of these moments took place rather late in his career, when he was in his fifties. At that time, even while he kept on with his practice in neurology and his more active interest in psychiatry, he had found himself attracted to the interaction between processes of law and what he termed "patterns of pathology that can pose a threat to other human beings." He had been asked by the Commissioner of Mental Health in Massachusetts to assist him in deciding how to ascertain the danger—and, more specifically, longevity of danger—represented by a person with a record of repeated physical assaults, typically on women, who had been arrested but whose legal disposition had yet to be resolved because there were questions about his psychiatric state.

Ethical, medical, and public safety factors frequently conflicted in these cases. Judges often found themselves bewildered in attempting to determine whether dangerous but psychiatrically disordered individuals ought to be considered knowledgeable actors in the crimes they had committed or whether, on the other hand, they should be perceived as mentally ill people who could not be held accountable for their behavior. In the latter situation, judges might assign them to a psychiatric institution, a secure facility operated by the state, with a sentence that was indeterminate in length.

The heart of the issue was the all-important question of a person's understanding of the "wrongness" of the crime he was committing, as well as the question as to whether the offender acted voluntarily or was under the compulsion of a force that he could not control. In order to evaluate the person's state of mind, the commissioner asked my father to become the director of a diagnostic center where evaluations could be carried out while psychiatric care could be provided in cases where my father felt that it was called for.

In a pattern of extensive preparation that had come to be familiar at other times in his career, my father began by looking at the research that existed on the questions he would now be facing. "The paucity of knowledge here in the United States," he wrote, led him "to begin by making a survey of the ways that other nations and societies had addressed the same dilemmas. I visited a variety of prisons and related institutions in the United Kingdom, Italy, France, the Netherlands, and Denmark," and "conducted colloquies with Swedish and Norwegian specialists." While he was in England, he said he'd made a point of "visiting the Institute of Criminology at Cambridge" and "spent some time at Broadmoor, the first of Britain's 'special institutions' for the criminally insane," from which he said he took away "both valuable and cautionary lessons."

All of this, the research he had carried out as well as the experience he subsequently gained in taking on the obligations he had been assigned by the commissioner, represent the background for a highly controversial case in which my father found himself recruited as an expert witness, not by the State of Massachusetts in this instance, but by the federal government. The case was that of Patricia Hearst, the daughter of the newspaper publisher William Randolph Hearst, who participated in an armed bank robbery after being kidnapped by a group of individuals who called themselves a "liberation army" and who justified their actions on the basis of a barely comprehensible political agenda.

Patricia was caught by a surveillance camera holding a weapon in her hands during the bank robbery, which took place in San Francisco in mid-April 1974. A month later, she was seen spraying bullets from a semiautomatic to give cover to escaping members of the "liberation army" after they had carried out a second act of robbery, this time in Los Angeles.

Following the deaths of six members of the group in a shoot-out with police, Patricia had gone underground with two other members and managed to elude police for sixteen months, until she was arrested in September 1975. A "self-employed urban guerilla" was the way that she identified herself when she was brought to jail.

In the trial that followed, Patricia's father retained a well-known lawyer by the name of F. Lee Bailey, who assembled a defense team that included a psychiatrist who had studied thought control and methods of brainwashing. The U.S. attorney who led the prosecution brought in two experts of his own. One of them—I remember that I had reacted to this with decidedly mixed feelings—was my father.

The reason this unsettled me, which I told him at the time, was that federal law officials and specifically the FBI had been engaged for several years in illegal and covert activities intended to subvert the social protest movements that had swept across the nation since the 1960s. The FBI had tapped the telephone of Dr. Martin Luther King and made recordings of his private conversations in an effort to discredit him, and it had harassed and attempted to incriminate others who were active in the civil rights and anti-war campaigns. (I myself had a lengthy dossier, which my lawyer obtained for me from the FBI and which reported on my civil rights activities and even on the lessons I was teaching in the 1960s in my fourth-grade class in Roxbury.) None of this, I realize, had any relevance at all to the very special case of Patricia Hearst and to the question of her guilt or innocence. My uneasiness with my father's role was a visceral reaction and was certainly not fair to him.

My father, in any event, agreed to be a witness in the case, although he made it clear that whatever testimony he would ultimately give was going to depend on his interpretation of the interviews he would need to have with the defendant and that he could not predict where those interviews would lead. Once he was assured that the prosecution understood the terms of his participation, he set aside his work in Boston for two months and flew to San Francisco to immerse himself in preparation for the trial.

Not in my father's desk, but in the metal filing case nearby, I had come upon the written records he had kept of his conversations with Patricia. I also found a transcript of his testimony and the cross-examination that he underwent at the hands of Mr. Bailey, who comes across as having been a rather less sophisticated litigator than his reputation would have led me to expect.

My father, after having spent sixteen hours with Patricia in five separate interviews, had come to the conclusion that she'd acted voluntarily, not under coercion, psychological or otherwise, in commission of the crimes of which she was accused. And while he commiserated with her for the situation in which she had found herself, his role was to assess the question of responsibility.

In his testimony to the court, he stated his opinion, based upon Patricia's answers to his questions and other interviews that were part of the court record, that she had grown up with an image of herself as, "in a sense, an abandoned child"—abandoned to the care of "a very harsh [and] arbitrary governess" at whose hands she reported that she had been beaten and otherwise mistreated. (My father emphasized that he was not stating these events as points of fact, because he had no firsthand knowledge of those years, but that these were the beliefs Patricia held or the impressions she conveyed.) She also spoke to him of fights between her parents and, while she indicated that these were purely verbal altercations, she said their quarrels had upset her so much that she wanted to leave home and asked to be sent away to a boarding school she had attended earlier. "She said," he testified, that "the only reason" she had done this was "to get out of that house."

While recognizing that many homes have problems of this nature, and being very careful not to demonize her parents, he nonetheless believed, not only for these reasons but also on the basis of emotional distress she'd undergone more recently— furious anger at a man with whom she had been living and had planned to marry but whose arrogant and chauvinistic manner and self-centered social values had upset her greatly—that she had, step by step, emerged into a state of mind, strong-willed and rebellious and hostile to authority, that rendered her receptive to the values of the people who had captured her.

An "embittered" person at the time when she was kidnapped, "angry…, unhappy…, ready to lash out," as he testified before the court, she was "a rebel in search of a cause." And "the cause," he argued, "found her."

In one of the most interesting portions of his testimony, my father described a classic exercise he'd carried out, in which he'd asked Patricia to draw a picture, essentially a "floor-plan," of the apartment in which her captors held her. Mr. Bailey, in his presentation, had spoken of "a closet" in which she'd been kept after being captured and the sense of terror this had caused, which, he argued, had reduced her to passivity. In the drawing, however, which indicated windows, a kitchen, a bathroom, and the like, Patricia had neglected to include the closet, which Mr. Bailey had described as one of the most traumatic focal points of her experience throughout this time and the fulcrum of the argument that she'd been tormented by her captors into a state of acquiescent desperation, which led her, once she had been freed from her captivity, to collaborate in violent behavior.

The absence of the closet from the drawing was of compelling interest to my father because it seemed to undermine the primary significance that Bailey had assigned to this experience, and it may have proven influential in the jury's judgment, reinforcing, as it did, other points my father raised, based on the conclusions he had drawn from talking with Patricia. In the strength of these conclusions, he was able to sustain the tough assault that Mr. Bailey launched upon his credibility.

Mr. Bailey badgered him, for instance, about his methods of note taking in his conversations with Patricia and asked him to explain why he did not tape-record these interviews. My father said it was not his practice to use a tape recorder in examinations. In the case of a defendant who has had the benefit of "eminent legal talent," he observed, "there is a high likelihood the person will be talking for the record," drawing upon "a memorized script" in which, as he implied, her lawyer would presumably have drilled her in advance. The presence of a tape recorder would intensify the likelihood that she would be sticking closely to that script and would thereby compromise "the integrity of the examination."

If he did not use a tape recorder, Mr. Bailey asked, what other method of recording did my father use? "You don't take shorthand, do you, Doctor?"

"No," my father said.

Mr. Bailey pressed the point. "What method *did* you use, please?"

"I used my right hand and a pen and a piece of paper right in front of me," my father said politely.

My mother, who was there throughout the trial, said that Mr. Bailey seemed to be unhappy with this answer.

In the end, what may have been the most decisive factor in the outcome of the trial was that Mr. Bailey, when he rose for his summation, could not focus on the points that mattered most in the exoneration of his client but rambled in perplexing ways that were difficult to follow—Patricia later said she wondered if he had been drinking—which, by any standard, represented a betrayal of her interests. Patricia was found guilty and given a long sentence, later reduced to seven years, of which she served somewhat less than two before President Jimmy Carter granted her a commutation.

In reading these materials, I was struck again, as I'd been in following the trial nearly thirty years before, by the poised and graceful way in which my father held his own in the give-and-take of cross-examination. Still, I remember I had been relieved when the case was over. His involvement in the trial, which had been given unrelenting press attention, placed him briefly in the public eye. And, in his obituaries, this event was treated as if it were emblematic of his life and his vocation, to the relative exclusion of his clinical career. I found this emphasis disheartening. Several of his former patients wrote to me expressing the same feeling.

It was now the spring of 2005, two years and six months since my father had come home to the apartment. Even though his hands were agile and he kept on making jottings on those pieces of blue paper when he was sitting at his desk with Julia, I noticed that, at bedtime, before he fell asleep, he would often curl his fingers into fists and hold them pressed against his chest.

As time went on, he did this more insistently. Silvia and Julia inserted pieces of soft towel underneath his fingers so that he would not do damage to his palms. If I spoke to him and stroked his fingers gently and he was alert enough to look at me directly, he would sometimes open up one of those hands and let me hold it in my own. As slight a thing as this may seem, I always took it as a little victory.

At the end of April, my father's trust attorney told me that my parents had exhausted their life savings. Their only income, from this date on, apart from the social security checks they would continue to receive, would be my father's very modest pension from the Massachusetts mental health department. This, the lawyer said, would meet their rental costs and some other items of a minor nature. The remainder of their costs—medical expenses not covered by insurance and not reimbursed by Medicare, as well as the costs of medically related needs such as special supplementary nutriments that both of them required, and, by far the largest item, salaries for their attendants—amounted to more than $15,000 monthly, or nearly $200,000 for each year that they remained alive.

The lawyer said he realized that my sister was in no position to assist in their support. She had, as I've noted, children of her own. They were grown-up women now, and both of them were married, but she tried her best to help them out, and she had other financial needs and obligations closer to her home. I already knew this. My situation was much simpler than hers.

The lawyer also said he needed to point out to me that, if I were willing to declare my parents indigent, which would call for selling off any of their physical belongings that had financial value, they would qualify for Medicaid, in which case the government would cover the expenses for my mother to reside within a nursing home, and for my father to return to one. But he also said he recognized that this was an option I would view as unacceptable. After having brought my father home at last, I could not imagine anything more disconcerting than to return him to an institution and, this time, my mother with him.

I naturally said nothing of this to my mother, but I know she had suspicions about what was going on, because Julia told me that she worried whether I was taking money from my own life savings and might later find myself in trouble if I lived as long as she and Daddy had. When one of my books landed, all too briefly, on the New York Times bestseller list in October of that year, Julia showed this to my mother to convince her that I wasn't on the verge of destitution. This quieted my mother's worries, Julia said, but only temporarily. "Then she would start in again....She'd question me repeatedly."

My mother had told Julia once that, during World War II, she had worked as "an investigator" (I don't think she ever said what she was investigating) for one of the branches of the military. She also said that she'd enjoyed this work tremendously. "I couldn't keep from smiling when she told me this," said Julia. "I said to myself, 'You better believe it! Once she knows she's on the track of finding something out, I don't think that anyone or anything can stop her.'"

I asked Julia recently about the question that had worried me before I brought my father home: Would my mother feel competitive with Daddy after she had been accustomed for so many years to the undivided and solicitous attention of her helpers?

"At first she *was* a bit competitive," said Julia. "If I was talking with her in her bedroom in the evening, I might look up at the clock and tell her that I had to go and give your father medicine. She'd say, 'Do you have to do it now?' When I'd tell her yes, it was important for your father, she would say, 'Well, hurry up! And do it fast! And then come back to me.'

"But after a while something changed. It got to the point where we'd be talking and she'd look up at the clock and tell me, 'Julia, I think it's time for you to go and get the medicine for Harry.'

"I'd say, 'Thank you for reminding me.' When I came back, she'd want to know if he had fallen asleep again and whether he was comfortable."

When my father first came home, as I have said, my mother started calling him "the baby." But after he'd been home some months, Julia told me she would sometimes speak of him more tenderly as "Harry."

"She'd go back and forth on this. Now and then, before she went to sleep, she'd decide she wanted to go in and look at him and see if there was any change. 'Julia,' she would say, 'take me to see Harry.' I'd help her to get out of bed and bring her to his room and I'd lower the guardrail on his bed and she'd kiss him on his forehead. After that, she'd stand there looking at him steadily...

"Then it was like a switch or something clicked within her mind and she'd say, 'Yes, he's still a baby.'" Julia said she was sure my mother didn't really think he was going to be any different one night from the night before. "I couldn't tell exactly what was going through her mind. Anyway, we'd be walking back into her bedroom and she'd say, 'No change. Still the same....' And that was the end of it."

Every so often, people who had known my father many years before would call and ask if they could speak to him. Or if they knew that he was ill,

Julia said they'd ask how he was doing. "One of the Chaplin girls has called up a few times," she said. "It was Victoria. The last time that she called was just about two weeks ago.

"She was in Boston for some reason and she wanted to come up and see your father. When I told her that I didn't think this was a good idea, she said she'd like to see your mother and she asked if she could take her out to lunch. Your mother took the phone and spoke with her and asked about her sisters, but she said she didn't think she had the strength to get dressed up and go out to a restaurant. Victoria asked if she could just come up and say hello. I was hoping your mother would agree, but she said she simply wasn't feeling well enough to have a visitor. I could tell Victoria was disappointed, but she told me that she understood."

My mother had told Julia once that she and my father had been invited back to Switzerland for the marriage of one of the Chaplin daughters, and she had described the wedding in the smallest details. "She said that it was at their home, and not in a hotel." Her memory of the daughters from the first time she had met them, Julia said, remained extremely clear. "One of them, your mother said, ran away from home when she was seventeen. Her boyfriend was an actor. She told me Mr. Chaplin was very angry with her when she did this, because she was so young, even though she said that he had married Mrs. Chaplin when she was a young girl too.

You know your mother. 'Serves him right!' I think that was Victoria....

"Anyway, I was sorry that your mother wouldn't let her come to the apartment. I think it would have done her good. I know how much she liked her."

Julia believed, as I did, that it was a matter of my mother's vanity. Every time she'd visited my father in the nursing home, she had gone with Julia to get her hair done at a place in Copley Square. Sometimes she had also gone to one of the stores nearby and bought herself a pretty dress, because she was "going out." Julia said my mother worried constantly about the way she looked because she said that she had never felt she was attractive. "Do you know, Julia," she had told her, "it's not an easy thing to be a woman and grow up to feel you're ugly."

She'd said something very much like that to me a long time before. When I had protested at her words, she told me my opinion did not count. "You're my son. All children want to think their mother's beautiful."

She was adamant about this.

During the last years of my mother's life— Julia described this after my mother died—the two of them had several conversations on the subject of religion. My mother would question her about her own beliefs and would ask about the church that she attended. Julia, like many of the mothers and grandmothers I had come to know when I was teaching in her neighborhood, was a devout believer. My mother's beliefs—not surprisingly, given her irreverent personality—were far more tentative and qualified.

I realize I've said almost nothing up to now about my mother's feelings or convictions on this subject—or those of my father, which, in honesty, should probably be called his absence of conviction or, to be entirely blunt about it, his vehement resistance to the tenets of conventional religion. (His Harvard thesis, it will be recalled, was titled "Religion and Insanity.")

After he and my mother had been married—in a nonreligious ceremony in a small town in New Hampshire—they had become members of a synagogue, but they attended services only intermittently, sometimes on a Friday night, mostly on the holy days. My father told me afterward that he remained a member of the synagogue primarily for social reasons—"in submission," as he put it, "to proprieties," but also out of his respect for his older brother, who was a leading figure in the congregation.

All of this was not without its complications and apparent contradictions. My father sent me and my sister to religious school once a week for several years, and he hired someone to come to our house for about six weeks one summer and try to teach me Hebrew before my bar mitzvah, but here again he gave me the impression that he did this as a matter of correctness in the face of social pressure. I don't know if there was more to it than that, but I didn't have the feeling that his motives were religious.

I think his attitude about religion might have been quite different if his mother's faith had been transmitted to him in a way that took deep roots within his heart, as it did (emotionally at least) for me, rather than, as he described it, "mostly as a lot of rules and dire threats that made no sense to me," which he'd rejected by the time he entered college. My grandmother (Bubee, as I called her) had somehow given me, on the evenings that I used to spend with her while I was in college, a less admonitory and more personally stirring sense of her religious faith than she had imparted to my father.

I knew he loved his mother deeply—he spoke about her as if she were still alive while he was in the nursing home—but I knew he'd also been afraid of her. He called her "the generalissimo" and said she was "a walking terror" when it came to Jewish people who did not obey the rules by which she lived. (He told me she had walked into a Chinese restaurant one night and, finding a member of her congregation eating ribs and shrimp and rice, she took his plate of food "and dumped the whole thing over him.")

It was my good fortune that she'd mellowed through the years and was more forgiving with her nonobservant grandson than she'd been with people of her generation or with her own children. But by this moment in her life, a gentleness and generosity pervaded everything.

My father's resistance never softened with the years, while my mother's independent disposition and the spiky nature of her character had led her to evolve her own original ideas about religion. She often told me she believed in God, not as some imaginable being who handed down a set of laws that Moses had transcribed while standing on a mountaintop—which she said that she regarded as "improbable"—but as a transcendent force, some kind of ethical but abstract entity, a benevolent presence in the world, as vague as that may be. She also said she was convinced there was a moral reason for our being, and she admired people who believed this and whose lives gave evidence of this belief.

This may be one reason why, when she was nearly ninety-eight, she began to question me insistently about one of my closest friends and colleagues in New York, an Episcopal priest named Martha Overall, the pastor of a congregation in the same impoverished South Bronx neighborhood where I was spending time with children and whom I'd described in detail in a book, Amazing Grace, which Julia had been reading with my mother. Martha's self-denying life and her devotion to the children in that neighborhood elicited a sense of reverence in my mother and she asked if I would bring the priest to visit her someday. Since Martha came to Massachusetts now and then for what are known as "pastoral retreats," she took one of these opportunities to come to the apartment and become acquainted with my mother.

This is how they got to meet each other and, because Martha had a maverick's spirit and a lot of independent values of her own, my mother's feisty personality appealed to her. She said that she enjoyed my mother's sense of humor, even the outrageously improper things my mother would allow herself to say with fewer and fewer inhibitions in the period when Martha got to know her.

Never proselytizing—it was not in keeping with her character to do so—Martha nonetheless discovered before long that she had been elected by my mother as her mentor in what she continued to believe to be the dubious idea of immortality, an idea that I think she somehow *wanted* to believe in, if not in the way a priest believes in this, then in some other way that she might find agreeable. The main point, though, is that she came to place tremendous faith in Martha's sense of ethical integrity. As a result, she asked her finally if, at the time when she passed on, Martha would conduct the service at her burial.

Martha has a seemingly unlimited compassion for the frailties or, more to the point in my mother's situation, the vulnerable uncertainties of others.

Her visits brought a quiet sense of reassurance to my mother in the face of the unknowable. Mostly, however, the two of them just had cheerful times together. Even in those final years when my mother wouldn't let Victoria or other old acquaintances come up to the apartment, Julia said that "she would ask me all the time when Martha would be coming back to visit her."

Martha, of course, never had to undergo my mother's crotchety and commandeering ways. My mother saved those tendencies primarily for me and for the patient women who took care of her while they also did their best to meet my father's needs and bring some joy into his life, as long as life remained to him.

CHAPTER TEN

My Mother Gives Me My Instructions

More and more, from that time on, as my father steadily declined into the condition of a very gentle, usually sleepy, and bewildered-looking little boy, my mother emerged in greater fullness and complexity.

Julia was with her in the evenings now more frequently than Silvia, who usually arrived at the apartment in the early morning and had to spend almost the entire day tending to my father. It wasn't until he went to bed, usually by six o'clock, that my mother had an opportunity for the company and conversation she enjoyed with Julia. In view of the many hours she and Julia spent with one another, I think I ought to say something, which I've avoided up to now, about the way in which my mother treated Julia.

When Julia had agreed to be my mother's

helper, there had been a question in my mind about the way my mother might behave with her. In the 1940s, when I was growing up, women of color were regarded by white women in the wealthier communities primarily as servants. Most of the families of my friends had a "colored maid"—or "colored girl," as it was generally said—to clean their homes and take care of their children. And, no matter how close they might come to be to one another (and the mothers of my friends talked incessantly, it seemed, about how much they loved their maids and how grateful to them they'd become), their relationships, of course, had been dramatically unequal.

My mother's relationship with Julia was unequal too. My mother remained the boss within her home; Julia had been hired to take care of her. But something had changed within my mother's attitude and understanding through the years. I've noted, for example, the kindness and affection she displayed to the children I would bring with me to visit her when I was a teacher. The civil rights era had a gradually transformative effect on both my mother and my father, and my direct involvement in the racial confrontations here in Boston had won my mother's strong support and, in time, my father's.

Still, Julia was not one of those little kids I used to teach, with whom it had been easy for a woman of my mother's race and class to empathize. I asked Julia, therefore, to be candid with me if, along with my mother's customary crankiness, she also picked up hints of any of those racially charged attitudes I remembered from my childhood.

"Don't worry," Julia told me, "I can take it. I grew up in the old days too. If I sense it, I'll know where it's coming from."

But I didn't *want* her to be obliged to "take it." So I felt a great sense of relief when Julia described to me the depth of the relationship that had evolved between them in those final years and, at a time of special need in Julia's life, the consolation and support my mother gave her.

"Your mother had a rare ability for someone of her age to put aside her own concerns when she could see that I was suffering. She tried so hard to comfort me when my husband died"—my father was in the nursing home when Julia's husband passed away—"and she talked with me for hours of 'the price we pay for love,' which was one of the ideas she kept returning to. When I needed to, I would cry in front of her. She would say, 'Pull up the chair. Sit right here beside me.' If I kept on crying, she would hold me in her arms. She was still so strong in spirit. I felt stronger when she spoke to me....

"If now and then she hurt my feelings, she would recognize it right away. 'I'm sorry, Julia,' she would say. If I'd gone into the living room, she would call to me. 'Julia, would you come back here to the bedroom? I need to apologize to you.'"

Perhaps the greatest cause of sorrow Julia underwent during those years was the profound depression of one of her grandsons and then his sudden suicide. She never recovered from that loss and, when she needed to unburden the emotions she was bearing and the sense of guilt that she was feeling, my mother, she said, would speak to her of other people she had known who had lost someone they loved to suicide and the way they blamed themselves for having been unable to prevent it.

"This helped me more than I can tell you," Julia said, "because I'd known, of course, that he was sick. He'd been away at college when he fell into depression. He couldn't keep on with his studies. He dropped out. I told him to come home and I would take him in to live with me.

"For a while after that, I thought that he was getting better. He'd been put on medication and he seemed to be more stable. Then, for some reason— I don't know why—he decided not to take his medicine. That was just before he killed himself. Even though I had no way to know this, I put the blame upon myself. I would tell this to your mother. She couldn't relieve me of the pain but she helped to take away the guilt that I was clinging to.

" 'Julia,' she would say, 'I understand a lot about depression. I will not allow you to believe this was your fault or your responsibility.' She was very firm with me...."

Julia underwent another painful loss when her mother died, two years before my mother's death. Again, she said, my mother put her own concerns aside. "She'd reach out for my hands and ask me to sit close to her. 'Julia,' she said, 'I know the loneliness you feel. You're going to miss your mother for a long, long time. But you'll be able to talk with me. I will be your mother now. I'll help you to get through this.' "

I was grateful to have heard these memories described in Julia's words. She was by now—I don't think this overstates the truth of things—probably my mother's closest friend and, certainly, most trusted confidante. The sense of loyalty between them was rock solid.

My mother was one hundred years old when Julia's mother died. Throughout that year and in the beginning of the year to come she continued to get out of bed each day to go into the living room to have her lunch, sometimes tea, and usually supper at the dinner table, and to go into my father's bedroom every night or two to stand there by his side, watching him in silence, then leaning down to kiss him. She remained clearheaded, for the most part, in her conversations with Silvia and Julia. If I visited on a night when she was in a cranky mood, she continued to be every bit as bossy and assertive with me as she'd always been.

One evening she studied the pin-striped shirt and dark blue necktie I was wearing. "I like that shirt...." She tested the fabric with her fingers. "I want you to buy more of them."

Another night she asked me, "Did you have a haircut?" I'd been working on a writing deadline and I hadn't had a haircut for more than a month, until the day before.

"Don't let it get too long again," she told me. "You look younger when it's short. Keep it that way!"

Julia, who was with us, couldn't keep herself from laughing. "Mrs. Kozol, you keep on surprising me!" Later, in the living room, Julia said, "Your mother does the same with me. If I'm wearing something new, she'll tell me that she likes it and she'll even ask me where I bought it, or how much I paid for it!"

During that year, my mother and I had a number of long and lively conversations in which, at my prodding, she would fill me in on details of her childhood and college years and the European visits she had made throughout the decades with my father. In the period when they had made their earliest transatlantic journeys, she told me that you couldn't make the trip by air. They traveled on old-fashioned steamships, packing their clothes in steamer trunks, which, she said, were fitted with drawers like those of a bureau. In one of her closets she still had a trunk like that, plastered with labels bearing the names of ships on which they'd sailed.

In subsequent years, when air travel to Europe came to be routine, they still preferred to travel on one of the famous liners of that era, the Liberté or Île de France or the old Queen Mary or a beautiful Italian liner called the Michelangelo. By the late 1950s and the 1960s, when my father's practice permitted them to stay in more expensive and more elegant hotels than in the past, she told me they stayed at places like the Hassler at the Spanish Steps in Rome or the Plaza Athénée in Paris.

One night, she told me of a dream she had in which she was sitting at a table in the lobby of the Plaza Athénée. "I was all alone. I don't know why. I think I was waiting for your father to arrive." She said her dream was full of questions about choosing the room where they would stay and where she'd put her passport and why my father was delayed. She said she sat there in the lobby waiting for three days.

On the third night my father arrived. At last she was able to go up to their room. My father was getting dressed for dinner—"a black-tie event," according to my mother. "He asked me to help him fix his tie." Then, she said, they went downstairs. A French physician and his wife were waiting for them "in a little funny-looking car" outside of the hotel.

"It seemed so real to me!" she said. She also told me that, while she was dreaming, she said to herself, "I think I've had this dream before...." She asked me if I'd ever had the same experience.

"Many times!" I told her. "I know I'm dreaming, but I keep on thinking, 'I've been in this place before.'"

"That's what it was like," she said. The odd experience of waiting in the lobby for my father to arrive was the only part that had unsettled her.

Another night, she told me more about the years when she was growing up in Dorchester, in a mostly Jewish neighborhood which, however, was adjacent to an area where many wealthy Irish people lived. "President Kennedy's mother, Rose Fitzgerald, lived about a mile from us in a neighborhood called Ashmont Hill. In the winter we would see her riding in a two-horse buggy with her father...."

"We had gas lighting in our house when I was born and there were gaslights on our street. A man who had a long pole would come on a bicycle and turn them on at night." She said she remembered how exciting it had been when electric lighting was installed.

Her father was a dentist and, she said, he had a busy practice by the time that she was born. He had been a member of the class of 1898 at Tufts University, to which he'd been admitted only two years after he'd arrived from Russia. Starting at about the age of ten, my mother used to go with him on Saturdays and help to clean his office and, if he had a Saturday appointment, she would stand beside him near the dental chair and hand him instruments he needed.

"We went together on the trolley. His office was on Tremont Street, near Jordan Marsh"—a well-known department store, now closed, that was a familiar landmark in the downtown business section of the city for more than a century.

My mother's father, who would live until the

age of ninety-two, continued with his dental practice up into his eighties. Grandpa, as I knew, had been an ardent socialist, but he never spoke to me of his political beliefs. He liked to talk about the books he read—nineteenth-century novels mostly, British and American. He had in his study a leather-bound edition of the novels of Charles Dickens. When I was eleven or twelve, he introduced me to The Pickwick Papers, Oliver Twist, David Copperfield, Hard Times, and Great Expectations. He would let me take them home to read on summer nights and later gave me the entire collection.

My mother's mother, who was a beautiful woman, had grown up in Budapest and had been steeped in the musical traditions of the end of the nineteenth century in Austria and Hungary. I remember, when I was five or six years old, listening to Nanny, as I called her, playing cheerful waltzes and light operatic music on the piano in her living room. It was she who had decided that my mother needed to take violin instruction, and my mother came to love the violin and regretted that she'd given up her lessons when she went to college.

Her early immersion in music, however, especially in chamber music, left behind an imprint that endured into her married years, as I remember from the time when I was starting elementary school and we had a phonograph—my mother called it "the Victrola"—on which she'd play the music she had come to know in childhood. Her favorite was a romantic piece, the piano quintet, opus 44, of Robert Schumann. She would sometimes hum its theme, introduced in the initial movement, while I was sitting with her in the kitchen.

After Latin School, my mother went to Wheaton, a small women's college about an hour south of Boston. Her parents moved from Dorchester to Brookline, a fashionable suburb, while she was in her freshman year at Wheaton. Her younger brother entered Harvard two years later. As it happened, he was in the same class as my father and, in time, invited him to come home to Brookline with him for a Sunday dinner, which is how my father met my mother.

They married while my father was in law school, secretly at first, because her mother looked down on my father's family, which was a great deal poorer and, from her genteel point of view, "less cultivated" than her own, which seemed, as far as I have ever learned, to be the only reason she opposed their getting married.

Daddy's mother, as he'd told me once, had her reservations too. "She worried whether it was wise for me to marry when I had so little money to support myself. But when I told her we'd already done it, that we'd been married in New Hampshire," and when they agreed to have a second ceremony in a rabbi's house to appease her sensibilities, "she accepted everything...."

Their honeymoon turned out to be the trip they

made to Switzerland in order for my father to obtain
the meeting he had sought with Eugen Bleuler. Elegant hotels were far beyond their budget in those
days. "We stayed in the most inexpensive inns that
we could find. We counted every penny that we
spent." It was, she said, "the happiest time in my
entire life. I was so proud of your father! And he was
so handsome!" She told me they would take long
walks along the lake when they were in Geneva.
"He used to wear one of those hats you see in the
old movies. He'd tip it to strangers as they passed."
When they arrived at the Burghölzli, which was Dr.
Bleuler's sanatorium in Zurich, "the doctor brought
us to his home, which was in a pretty town outside of
the city. He insisted that we stay and dine there with
him and his family!"

My mother said they stayed in Zurich longer
than they'd planned because of Dr. Bleuler's graciousness to Daddy. "He invited him to sit in on
consultations and go with the other doctors when
they were examining the patients." Once, while
Daddy was preoccupied with these observations,
"Dr. Bleuler took me off to see the different neighborhoods of Zurich." At the end of the day, she said,
"he took me to an ice cream parlor and he bought
me chocolate ice cream. He was an elderly man by
then, but he was so kind to me! When I dropped my
handkerchief, before I could pick it up, he stooped
down and handed it to me."

When Dr. Bleuler learned that they were on

their honeymoon, he told them about other places that he thought they ought to visit while they were in Switzerland. "We went to Interlaken. We traveled on the little boats that went across the lakes. We took one of those tiny trains that went right up the mountainsides. We spent a few days in Lausanne. Then to go to Paris and to meet Pierre Janet! Can you imagine how exciting all of this had been for me?"

Their marriage, however, as I knew, had not been consistently idyllic—nor, to put a finer point on this, anywhere near as perfect as I had, like many children, wanted to believe when I was growing up. Only a few months after she had spoken so nostalgically about those weeks in Switzerland, my mother startled me by letting me in on a secret that she said she'd never shared with anyone before. She told me she had fallen in love with two other men during her years of marriage, the first time in her early thirties, only eight years after she'd been married, the second time when she was in her forties.

The first of these men, whose name was Benedict Alper, had been my father's closest friend in college. Ben had been a charming and good-looking man who cut a dashing and romantic figure and whose family had sufficient wealth to enable him to own a car—it had a "rumble seat," my mother said—which he sometimes let my father use when he began to court her. She became much closer to Ben during a period of loneliness she underwent when Daddy was a resident at the Boston Psychopathic and had to be away from home as long as six weeks at a time.

It was all the harder for her, she confessed, because she knew my father was attracted to "the pretty nurses" (my mother's words) who worked beside him at the hospital and with whom, as she suspected, he allowed himself more than a few flirtations and, as she would later learn, more than mere flirtations.

She wanted me to know that her relationship with Ben had never become sexual, but she gave me the impression she would not have minded if it was. She said she didn't think Ben ever guessed how strongly she was drawn to him.

The second time she had "betrayed" my father— that was the word she used—things had gone much further. "I had a love affair," she said, not at all remorsefully but in a voice of thrilling secrecy. She didn't tell me the name of the man and she made it a point to tell me that, despite this episode of infidelity and the pain my father caused her by his own more frequent acts of indiscretion, she had never ceased to love him deeply and to take tremendous pride in his career. All in all, looking back, she said, she was glad that she had married him.

I could not resist the urge to ask her if she felt no guilt at all in thinking back upon her infidelity.

"Not a bit!" she said. "He did it. So did I." Abruptly, as was her habit, she brought the subject to an end. "Go into the other room and check up on the baby...."

That was not the last time my mother would surprise me by the candor and the tartness of her words. On another evening, early in December, when Julia was away and Silvia was sitting with me at my mother's bedside and my mother seemed to have been drifting off, perhaps into one of the fantasies or daydreams she increasingly enjoyed, Silvia and I fell into a conversation of our own. A gregarious woman, and highly inquisitive, Silvia had come to know quite a lot about my private life and my career, but she was always curious to learn a little more.

She said she knew from looking at my books that I got a lot of pleasure out of spending time with children when I visited their schools. "Do you ever wish," she asked, "that you had children of your own?"

My mother, as far off and distracted as she had appeared, was not as lost in daydreams as I had believed. The minute Silvia asked me about children, my mother's eyes were open wide. I hesitated briefly. Then I answered Silvia that it was, in fact, one of my real regrets that I had no children, but I said I didn't think it likely I'd be having children now, at this point in my life. This, as I probably could have guessed, was guaranteed to set my mother off.

"You can still have them! You're not too old."

"First we'll have to find a wife for him," said Silvia.

My mother looked at her with irritation. In a snappish voice, she asked her, "Why?"

"Mrs. Kozol!" Silvia said. "A man can't just go off and start out having babies if he hasn't bothered to find someone that he wants to marry!"

"That's absurd!" my mother said. "Why not?"

Silvia, the most conservative of women, who exercised the strictest discipline upon her daughter and granddaughter, looked aghast.

"Mrs. Kozol!" she said again. "What are you saying to your son?"

"That's the craziest thing I've ever heard," my mother said.

I don't think my mother actually believed what she had said in arguing with Silvia. But the words that bubbled up when she had risen to the battle against Silvia's respectability, as well as the story of the love affair she had belatedly revealed, opened up the vista of a ribald sense of moral independence in my mother that went further than I'd ever seen in her before.

Still, in spite of unexpectedly delicious moments like the one when she incited Silvia to wrath, it was apparent by the end of winter that my mother recognized a steepening decline in her clarity of thinking and the capability for detailed recollection in which she had taken so much pride.

"I'm beginning to lose my memory," she announced to me one night. "Sometimes there's a place that I remember. I can *see* it, but I can't think of the name."

"That happens to everyone," I said, wanting to reassure her. I asked her, on an impulse, whether she could call to mind any of the Latin words she'd learned during her high school years. Forgetting the concern she'd just expressed about her loss of memory, she replied by chanting out the entire conjugation of the first verb generations of young people used to learn in Latin class.

"Amo, Amas, Amat, Amamus, Amatis, Amant..."

"Excellent!" I said, as if we were back in school and I was the teacher. I asked if she remembered any nouns, and she declined "puella" (girl) in singular and plural. Maybe the fear attached for her, as for many students, to the first intimidating weeks of Latin class had locked this in her memory.

But the truth of the matter is that my mother's own assessment of her declining faculties was proving to be more accurate with every passing day. By the spring of the year, her appetite was waning and, more and more, she wouldn't eat the meals that Julia would insist on bringing to her bedroom. "Mrs. Kozol," Julia would say, "you need to eat some food." My mother, said Julia, would reply, "I don't *have* to. You can't make me. Take the tray away!" An hour later, she might call her back into the room and look at her scoldingly. "Julia, you didn't give me dinner!"

By May, however, even those brief stirrings of cantankerous vitality had become less frequent. Julia also noticed that she didn't ask so many questions about Daddy anymore. "Sometimes," Julia said, "it seemed as if she had forgotten he was still there in the room right next to hers...."

One night in June, my mother whispered to me something that I couldn't understand because she spoke so softly. When I leaned a little closer, she said there was something that she had to tell me, but she asked me first to go and close the door "so nobody can hear."

After I had shut the door and came back to sit with her, she said, "I have a lot of money right here in my purse." During the past year or so, she had taken to keeping a small pocketbook beside her in her bed, hidden usually beneath the blankets. She took it out and showed me that it held $200. "There's more in the bureau, underneath my sweaters. It's in the bottom drawer."

She kept speaking in a whisper. "If there's anything you need, I want you to have it. That's why I've kept it safe for you."

I realized she believed $200 was a large amount of money, as it would have been, of course, when she was a child. I didn't say a word that might have contradicted this impression. "I'm doing okay right now, Mom," I told her. "But if I need it sometime, I'll remember that it's here."

"It's my money. I'm your mother. I have the right to give it to anyone I want."

JONATHAN KOZOL

"I know you do. I won't forget," I promised her.

"Come here," she said.

After she had kissed me and I kissed her back, she said it was okay for me to go and open up the door. When she said she'd like "a little tea…, maybe some cheese," I went into the other room and Julia and I arranged things on a tray, three cups, one for each of us, and some Camembert and Emmenthal, still my mother's favorites. She still enjoyed a cup of tea—"not too strong," as she always said to Julia—but she barely nibbled at the cheese.

With the arrival of summer, my mother grew increasingly withdrawn from Silvia and Julia. When I was in her room alone with her, she sometimes managed to find sufficient strength to talk with me—no longer, however, in that commandeering way in which she used to issue her decisions and demands, but in a quieter, more passive tone, and usually only a few words at a time. Little by little, she began to say good-bye to me.

"I don't want you to be scared," she said to me one evening, holding my hand closely. "I'm not afraid to die. I want you to be strong. When it's time for me to go…" She didn't finish with the sentence.

As the summer went on, my mother's somewhat rigidified posture and more frequently closed eyes made it apparent that she was giving up the will to live even while she seemed to keep on fighting back against that loss of will. Her hands curled into tightened fists, not unlike the way my father held his hands, but in his situation it seemed to be a reflex action, without intentionality, while in my mother's case those fists took on a more embattled look, like those of someone getting ready for a last encounter that she knew she would not try too hard to win.

Even now, a sweet nostalgia and some of the mildest streams of memory from her early childhood appeared. She started to recite a rhyme her mother might have taught her in her infancy.

> One two
> Three four
> Five six seven
> All good children
> Go to Heaven....

She began by saying this only once or twice each time. Soon, however, she would say it maybe six or seven times without leaving any interruptions in between. It ceased to sound as if it gave her a consoling feeling. It became more automatic and mechanical.

By September, I noticed that her head was almost always tilted back when I came in the room. Her jaw had stiffened. Her mouth was generally open. Her fingers remained tightened into fists but did not look like those of someone who was fighting or resisting anymore. She rarely looked directly at me now unless I leaned across her body so that her upward-gazing eyes would meet my own.

When the time for which she had prepared me finally arrived—it was late October now—I knew I had my orders from my mother. I did not disobey her.

Swallowing difficulties and an aspiration problem caused by the flowing up of secretions from her stomach, or of undigested particles of food, into her throat and lungs, brought my mother into the hospital with severe congestion and with a low fever, which, however, worsened somewhat by the time she was examined and they got her upstairs into Phillips House. Antibiotics, I was told, might bring down the fever, but the aspiration problem, according to the resident, could only be addressed by insertion of a feeding tube into her stomach and a breathing tube into her throat.

"I don't think you want to do that to your mother at this stage of things," he said.

Looking at my mother's upturned face, her eyes closed, her mouth open, the hardened outline of her jaw, I stood by her bed and briefly examined the DNR when one of the nurses brought it to me for my signature. After I signed it, I stayed to watch the resident setting up the morphine drip. Julia stayed there with me at the bedside.

My mother remained alive for several hours.

When, as the first rays of the sun began to filter through the window shades, I heard her groaning once, I asked the resident if he could raise the morphine level. An hour later, he came in and did it once again. In the final moments, the nurse who had been present left the room, as Julia also did without my asking her. I wanted to be there by myself to give my mother one more hug and one good final kiss.

My mother had said she did not want a funeral but preferred a graveside ceremony. Lucinda and Julia and other people who had helped to care for her, and my sister and her daughters, a small number of relatives, and some of my closest friends who'd known my mother well, gathered at the grave site at Mount Auburn Cemetery. Martha read a passage from the Book of Ruth and spoke of my mother's character and of her long and interesting life in a quiet, contemplative service that I think she would have liked. On a CD player I had asked one of my friends to bring, we played the Schumann piano quintet, the passage in which a cellist and a violinist play that hauntingly romantic melody I knew my mother loved.

After the service I went back to the apartment, where Silvia had stayed in order to let Julia be present at the burial. My father was lying down in bed. His eyes were open. He was smiling. He had, of course, no understanding of the reason for my mother's absence if he even had an inkling of the fact that she was no longer in the room next door.

I went into my mother's room and looked at the photos on her bureau. The Red Sox jersey had been folded on a table near her bed. The purse that she had kept beside her was still there, partially hidden underneath the blankets. She had neglected to bring it with her when she went into the hospital.

CHAPTER ELEVEN

The Pursuit of Recollection

After my mother's death I continued to have conversations with her for a while. I would lie in bed at night and tell her what was going on within my life—something of interest that had taken place that day, a difficult decision I would have to deal with when I woke up the next morning. For more than a year, with a stubbornness I may have learned in part from her, I would not accept that I had lost her.

My father's trust attorney set up a meeting with me soon after the burial. He said that, with my mother's passing, it made even less sense than before to keep on paying rent for the apartment. He suggested again that Daddy's belongings ought to be sold off, so that the money paid for them could be applied to his expenses and exhausted quickly.

At that point, he would qualify for Medicaid and, as the lawyer said, we might find "a reasonably pleasant place" for him to stay for whatever time he might remain alive.

"You could save yourself a barrel of money, old boy," he observed, speaking, as always, in a patrician tone that made me think of the aristocratic boys from Groton and St. Paul's School I had known in college.

I don't think he actually believed his argument would be convincing to me. I'd already told him I had brought my father home because he had asked for this repeatedly. Whether or not he recognized it anymore, this was his home and I resolved that he would go on living here until he closed his eyes for the last time.

In the months after my mother died, the circadian rhythms of my father's life continued to be pretty much the same as they had been. "When I come in at seven," Silvia said, "I always say, 'Good morning, Dr. Kozol!' He looks right up at me, bright and alert. If he's lying on his side and facing my direction, he moves his eyes to follow me.

"If his eyes are closed when I bring his breakfast, I tell him, 'You have to open your eyes. I'm not going to give you breakfast if you keep them closed.' He obeys me! He opens them. Then when he sees me dip the spoon into the pudding or the applesauce, he opens his mouth and watches as I lift the spoon. After I put the food in his mouth, I see him chewing, even though he doesn't have to chew. He does it automatically....

"He loves puddings—anything sweet. His favorites are banana pudding, peach purée, mango pudding, and vanilla custard. I know this because he swallows them more quickly. When I give him a purée of vegetables, he takes it in his mouth but holds it there much longer."

Although his legs were very weak, his arms had remained strong, and he continued putting up a strenuous resistance when Silvia was bathing him. "He still would put his fists across his privates. No matter how many times I'd lift them up, he'd put them back again. Once, when I got really mad, I told him, 'Take those hands away!' He looked around sideways, since I was behind him, and he said, 'Oh my God!' And I told him, 'Good! I made you talk!'"

When I kissed him in the evenings now, he no longer had the strength to kiss me back. But he would press his lips against my cheek and sometimes he would just look up and study my face, as it seemed, with the greatest curiosity. That wonderful smile in his clear blue eyes that I had always loved would suddenly appear.

One of the bright young research aides who had worked with me a couple years before and still liked to visit with my father, and always brought him flowers to cheer up his room, noticed that the Boston Globe continued to arrive at the apartment every day. She was a bit perplexed by this because she knew he couldn't read it and would certainly no longer understand it even if Silvia were to read some stories to him.

I explained to her that I was trying to do everything I could to keep the environment around my father as civilized, familiar, and connected to the outside world as possible. The arrival of the paper and its presence on his desk or on a table in his bedroom was simply a small part of this. (Julia and Silvia, who was staying overnight now almost as frequently as Julia, would read it in the evenings once he fell asleep.) One of the final things I did after my father died was to cancel the subscription.

In the following year, my father had to go into the hospital again. The problem had begun in February when his geriatrician, in the course of an examination, discovered what she termed a "superficial ulcer," essentially an aggravated bedsore, just above his rectum. But she proposed no treatment for the ulcer and she set up no appointment for a follow-up exam. Instead, she said the visiting nurse would come to see my father on a weekly basis and would tell her promptly if the ulcer did not heal. But, as the ulcer failed to heal and progressively grew larger, the visiting nurse did not appear. The message from the doctor, for whatever reason, hadn't been conveyed to her.

By March 16, the ulcerated area had doubled in size and become what is known as "a necrotic abscess." The doctor later said, "It had been my impression that the...nurse and [a] wound care specialist had been following the patient closely...," but it seemed she hadn't taken any measures to be sure that this had been the case.

On March 17, another nurse appeared at the apartment. As soon as she looked at my father's wound, she said he should be taken to the hospital. A doctor told me late that night that a CAT scan had confirmed a "sacral ulcer with necrotic tissue" that might already have expanded well into his rectum. A surgeon, he said, had been called in for a consultation and antibiotics had been prescribed and were being given to my father through an intravenous line.

That night and the next three days I spoke or met with a series of physicians. The second physician told me that my father now was running a high fever and that he believed the abscess had, indeed, spread into his rectum. If this was so, there would be two options. "The extreme response would," he said, "be major surgery under anesthesia," which, he continued, "can be very difficult. He could die on the operating table." The alternative, he said, was that the infection might be arrested by the antibiotic medication my father was receiving and that he "might be relieved" and the abscess might begin to heal if he could be given proper care at home.

The following day, a different physician said that there appeared to have been no infection of the rectum, as was previously feared, and that my father's fever had come down. But the day after that, yet another doctor told me that the ulcer had been left untreated for too long and permitted to expand to so large a size that it was uncertain whether it would ever close—or not at least for many months, perhaps for an entire year.

In the face of these differing opinions, and without my father's regular physician (the "attending physician," as she was termed) to pull it all together and present me with a clear and understandable prognosis, I didn't know what I should do or which of these opinions I ought to rely upon. It was Silvia, in her unbounded confidence that she could help my father to recover sooner than the doctor said was probable—by which I mean the latest in the series of four doctors I had talked to—who swept away my sense of indecision and confusion and persuaded me to bring my father home as soon as this was possible.

Once he was at home, she and Julia set out on a course of action to protect the wounded area from further irritation by ordering a special kind of soft and cushioned mattress and positioning my father so that he was lying on his side when he was asleep, and not putting pressure on his rectum and his lower back. That was not an easy job. They had to watch him through the night, but they did it with painstaking care and the ulcer started healing.

As a matter of record, nonetheless, as Julia noted pointedly, my father's doctor "had been unavailable to us at the time we needed her." In view of this pattern, which was now predictable, friends have asked me why I didn't spare myself, and Silvia and Julia, from more of these frustrations by asking for advice from one of the physicians in the Boston area with whom I was acquainted in the hope that he could help me find another doctor for my father. I did, in fact, put out some inquiries, but I was advised that it wasn't likely any other doctor would be inclined, or think it wise, to intercede in my father's care at this stage in his life.

To start all over with a new physician would, in any case, destabilize the modus operandi to which Silvia and Julia had managed to accommodate themselves, no matter at how large a cost to their emotional endurance. The working relationships they had developed with some of the people in the doctor's office, who, as they said, sometimes were responsive and did get answers back to them without worrisome delays, would have to be entirely reconstructed with a new physician. Then too, it seemed, every time I thought of ending the relationship with my father's doctor, she would send me an extremely thoughtful ex post facto summary of his condition in the aftermath of one of these crises—highly detailed and, at times, almost apologetic—which would lead me to believe, temporarily at least, that she would be watching him more closely.

In the end, I decided not to try to make a new arrangement, even if I could have found one that was a significant improvement. Instead, I did the best I could to back up Silvia and Julia in the valiant efforts they were making to navigate a system of heartbreaking and bureaucratized medical impersonality for which, one can only hope, even in the face of currently disturbing trends, a more effective and humane alternative is someday put in place.

In the final twelve months of my father's life, as I saw him falling even further into the condition of an almost wholly passive, usually smiling, but totally dependent child, I looked for consolation and distraction once again by spending the late evening hours looking through the boxes of materials he had entrusted to me. In one of the cartons in which he'd filed copies of his correspondence and some printed papers from the years when he began his practice, I came upon a bold critique that he had written on the state of psychiatric education as he had observed it when he did his year of study at Johns Hopkins under Adolf Meyer.

The document, which he wrote only three years later, surprised me by the harshness of the language he had used in his evaluation of the teaching practices established by Meyer himself. (It surprised me all the more because, in the same package, there was a commanding portrait of Meyer, dedicated by the doctor "to my friend and pupil Dr. Harry Kozol," which my father had valued enough to have had it beautifully framed and which he had hung on his office wall next to a portrait signed by Dr. Bleuler.) The critique was presented in the form of a letter solicited by a physician named John Whitehorn who had been selected to take over the directorship of Dr. Meyer's clinic in the summer of 1941, when, as the letter indicates, Meyer was getting ready to retire.

"Dear John," the letter began. "I am sending you the report I promised.... I will direct your attention to the matter of the education of your medical students, about which I have not had much to say before. I shall take up the matters under different headings."

Under the first heading, "A Criticism of the Course Given by Dr. Meyer," my father had started off, unapologetically, "He overemphasized his own system and its various minutiae. This involved much memorization of his concepts of integration, psychobiology, etc. The students gained no perspective about psychiatry in general...." Whatever reference to the work of his contemporaries he presented at the morning meetings was "slight in nature and somewhat derogatory." This, my father contended, had a "boomerang" effect in that, later, "many of these same students grew so intrigued by psychoanalytic and other exploratory concepts" that "they went off the deep end," dismissing Dr. Meyer's concepts altogether.

Under the heading of "Relationship of the Phipps Clinic to Other Divisions of the Johns Hopkins Hospital," my father began, "The Phipps Clinic was in a psychological Siberia. There was very little intercourse between the psychiatric and medical divisions. This isolation was emphasized by the fact that it [the clinic] had its own medical internist, thus making it independent of the rest of the hospital. Not only was this insulting to the hospital, but it was also grossly unfair to the patients, because the quality of the medical consultation in the clinic itself was vastly inferior to what was available in the regular medical divisions of the hospital."

In reference to "The Regular Wards," my father said, "I do not think the patients got as thorough treatment as they ought to have received," because of an absence of proper supervision. "There was virtually never an instance of [a member of the senior staff] sitting down with a patient and the intern for an hour or even half an hour of careful questioning. The essential point is that the interns need to get some personal clinical teaching…, rather than second-hand discussion in the morning conferences based on their descriptions of what they think they have elicited from the patient.…

"Most of the training revolved around the morning meetings. Dr. Meyer would make sage comments after the intern read a long hand-written description of a patient's case. These [the meetings] were sometimes quite ridiculous in that the battle would revolve around a diagnosis but did not affect the treatment of the patient one way or the other....

"Although the supporters of the old regime will undoubtedly hotly deny it," he continued, "the interns gained virtually no experience in the handling of acute problems, such as combative deliria, wild manias, etc."

The thoroughness of patient care was also compromised, my father wrote, by poor organization in assignment of the interns. "The newly admitted patient would receive a great deal of attention for a week or two until his work-up was complete. After that, he would be dropped almost like a hot cake because the intern would be busy with other new admissions or would be distracted by a number of time-wasters. Thus, the patients would have quite a letdown in their third or fourth weeks in the clinic. After that, their meetings with the interns were usually brief and few."

Under the heading of "Laboratories," he had written, "I have virtually no comment. I see little point in making much of the anatomy lab, because it was a personal indulgence of Dr. Meyer. He stressed anatomy [but] with very little conception of physiology...."

Under the heading of "Psychoneuroses," he had written this: "The treatment and instruction in handling psychoneuroses has been one of the weakest points [in the clinic's operation]. I suggested to Dr. Meyer that a special division for the treatment of psychoneuroses over a long period of time ought to be established, but to no avail. In this respect, I think the clinic has fallen down in its responsibilities to American psychiatry."

In a final "Addendum re Psychoanalysis," my father proposed that the clinic might anticipate, and thereby prevent, the later rejection of all Meyerian ideas on the part of interns who were being given no exposure to non-Meyerian positions if it were to find "a refugee of eminence" who had been immersed in the psychoanalytic schools of Europe. "Up here [i.e., in Boston]," he went on, "we have a very able fellow, unbelievably dynamic...," whose experience included "the directorship of Freud's outpatient department for a great many years." After giving the name of the man he recommended, he added this description: Although "orthodox" in his beliefs, "he is not a stereotypical copy of Dr. Freud....He is always alert and contemplative" with "a rapier-like quickness of thinking, which is exceedingly stimulating....It might be a good idea to meet him and size him up yourself."

The doctor to whom these proposals were addressed replied to my father in what I thought, given the severity of my father's words, was a gracious note of thanks for "your very helpful and thoughtful letter." I have no idea if my father's recommendations had any consequence at all in policies established by the new director. I do know my father continued to maintain a close association with other doctors on the staff for many years to come.

In a larger and much later body of materials, dating from the 1960s, when he was evaluating criminal offenders who had been remanded to his care by the mental health department here in Massachusetts, I came upon another instance of my father's willingness to incur the risk of causing some discomfort for his colleagues or immediate superiors. It may seem surprising that I hadn't thought about this episode from so many years before until I was reminded of it now, because the story that unfolded from these documents had been of great importance to the public while it was taking place and remained a matter of contentious disagreement for several years thereafter.

The story began in 1962 and continued through 1963 and into 1964, when thirteen women, some of them elderly, one as old as eighty-five, were strangled in their homes in, or close to, Boston. Their bodies, according to a press account, were "strangely manipulated sexually," their "swollen necks garishly decorated with large, looping bows." A massive search was immediately begun for the single individual who, police believed, had probably carried out these strangulations on his own, but, as of 1965, no suspect had been found.

In that year, a patient at a large state mental hospital and prison complex, to which my father's treatment and evaluation center was attached, indicated to another patient that he was the one who had killed these women and, soon after, made a full confession to his lawyer, then to the state's attorney. The credibility of his confession was, however, clouded by the fact that the man had a seemingly compulsive inclination to outrageous braggadocio and appeared to be possessed of a desire to inflate his own importance, even in this instance by confessing to a crime that carried the potential punishment of life imprisonment or execution. (Massachusetts still permitted executions at that time.)

As in other cases in which there were questions about a suspect's psychiatric status, the court requested that my father help it to determine if the man in question had the mental competence to be brought to trial. My father subsequently interviewed the suspect, a former handyman and construction worker named Albert H. DeSalvo who already had a dossier of sexual assaults, none of which, however, had involved an act of murder.

The transcript of the interviews—which are dated March 14, 24, and 29, 1965—runs for 145 pages. Another psychiatrist sat in on the interviews, but his participation seems to have been minimal. In a cover letter submitted to the State Commissioner of Mental Health, my father noted that DeSalvo (whom he referred to as "the patient," rather than "the suspect") was "essentially responsive" to his questions but displayed the indications of "a state of shallow affect."

In these interviews, my father asked DeSalvo to describe the murders, which he did in rather gruesome detail but with no perceptible emotion and often with a choice of words that seemed to indicate he looked upon these strangulations as unfortunate events that had "happened" to these women as opposed to acts he had himself committed.

In speaking of one of the women whom he claimed that he had murdered, for example, DeSalvo told my father, "She was the one with the pillow case." My father noted the detachment of this phrasing from any indication that DeSalvo was connected somehow with the uses of that pillowcase. The pillowcase was "there." But how did it get there?

"What do you mean by that?" my father asked.

Only when so prompted did DeSalvo introduce himself into that portion of the narrative. "I used the pillow case on her" and "tied a knot" [i.e., around her throat], he finally said.

In another instance, he remarked of a woman who, he said, was in her sixties, "She died, fractured skull and stabbed."

"Who gave her the fractured skull?" my father asked.

"I did," said DeSalvo.

Again, in the case of a woman who had been in bed when he claimed that he had "slipped the lock" to enter her apartment, he said that "she got out of bed…" and "something strange…I don't know how to explain the feeling that came over me, looking at her.…And she turned and she was getting up and all I remember is her lyin' on the floor.…Stocking was around her neck."

My father had to ask him how the stocking got there, at which point DeSalvo said, "I put it there."

In some cases, DeSalvo told my father, he could not remember someone he had killed, or had no knowledge of exactly what he'd done, until he read about it in the paper. Only then did he become aware (my father's words) "that he had been the one who did the killing.…" His repeated references to newspaper accounts, as my father noted, raised the possibility, admittedly a faint one, that DeSalvo, who appeared to him as being very shrewd, inventive, and intelligent, might be manufacturing portions of these stories out of the plenitude of details that the newspapers were running, although other portions of the narrative did not awaken this suspicion.

In any event, if DeSalvo was in fact the perpetrator of these strangulations, my father recognized "a notable experiential unreality" within the man's perception of events he was describing. He remarked again upon the absence of emotion when DeSalvo spoke about the victims while at the same time conveying "an almost grandiose enjoyment of the fact that he was now the focus of great interest and consideration." These impressions, reinforced by other indications of irrationality and "a nearly absolute insensibility as to the endangerment in which he'd placed himself" by his confessions, led my father to believe the man should not stand trial.

"Albert H. DeSalvo," he wrote in his conclusions, "is suffering from a committable mental disease," as defined by Massachusetts law, with "grossly defective judgment," "lack of competence to comprehend his situation," and inability "to make decisions which will best serve his interest...."

My father's opinion was overruled, however, by others in the mental health department, who diagnosed DeSalvo as a schizophrenic but, at the same time, told the court that he was not insane and that he was capable of knowing right from wrong, a position that my father felt was legally and psychiatrically untenable.

The media, meanwhile, which already had adjudged DeSalvo to be guilty, was demanding he be brought to trial. The court at last decided that DeSalvo could be tried, not, however, for the thirteen strangulations but only for his earlier offenses, which, as I have noted, did not eventuate in homicide— a decision that my father viewed as "utterly illogical" and "inherently self-contradictory" and possibly tainted by political considerations.

The trial nonetheless went forward and resulted in an outcome that my father said was easily predictable. A jury that could not conceivably have been unbiased by exposure to the media—amazingly, the judge did not require that the jury be sequestered—found DeSalvo guilty on all charges. He was given a life sentence, taken from the hospital, and sent to a state prison, where no treatment was provided for his mental illness.

A year later, DeSalvo wrote a letter to my father from the penitentiary. The letter, which has never been made public but which my father had secured in a sealed envelope, was written by hand on sheets of blue-lined notebook paper and bears the date of January 1, 1968.

"Dear Dr. Kozol," DeSalvo had begun. "I have tried in vain to do what I felt was right. But for some unknown reason I find I'm at a stand-still. I have thought of you many times and can't understand why I never saw you again [i.e., after he was transferred from the hospital]. At least you showed me you were interested in me as a person and...I respect you very much for this."

He went on to say he thought my father "understood" what he was feeling. "I wanted very much to talk with you *alone*," he said, "and release everything inside me. I can't explain why, all I know is I felt so at ease with you....

"It's a shame you were not Medical Director"—a reference to the fact that another doctor, to whom my father was officially subordinate, was the one DeSalvo had to deal with for most of the period while he was under observation. If it had been otherwise, "all of what has happen[ed] could have been avoided. If you think about it you will realize what I mean."

After saying again that, in his present situation, he found himself "unable to release what's inside me," the man who had allegedly strangled thirteen women ended politely, "I hope this letter finds you in good health. Have a happy New Year."

In a postscript, crowded at the bottom of the page, he said he hoped my father would remember that he had "walked into the police station" on his own some years before and had asked for medical help. "And this," he said, "is the results.... I just don't understand." Five years later, still in prison, DeSalvo was murdered by another inmate. No other person ever went to trial for the strangulations.

In the folder that contained DeSalvo's letter, I came upon a memo that my father wrote, in which he again took issue with the doctors who had testified that DeSalvo was a schizophrenic but nonetheless was not insane and was capable of knowing right from wrong.

"In light of the absence of emotion," my father wrote, "and the sense of unreality that he conveyed in description of his crimes, the term schizophrenia would probably apply, because of the apparent fragmentation of his anima. But to attribute ethical perceptions—the recognition of good or evil, right or wrong—to a man with this division in his soul is a very loose and unconvincing formulation....

"DeSalvo was not capable of knowing right from

wrong if, by 'knowing,' we mean something more than recognizing, as a generality, that there exists a socially accepted set of values but, rather, knowing in a way that penetrates the essence of one's being and can therefore countermand an impulse or compulsion to take actions that will do grave damage to another human being. Any other kind of knowledge is inert, an ineffectual abstraction. In order to know, we have to feel. Without that capability, our knowledge has no value and no meaning."

The same assertiveness with which my father stated these beliefs, as well as the incrementally accelerating pace by which he made his argument and his agility in seizing on exactly the right words to encapsulate his meanings, remained the hallmarks of his writing for the rest of his career. Admittedly, along with his assertiveness, there was also that persistent inclination, when he took issue with another doctor, to express his disagreement in a manner that approached the adversarial. My mother used to worry that it wasn't in his interest to antagonize so many of his colleagues. "But this," she said, "was part and parcel of his personality. His mother, I don't need to tell you, could be hard on other people too. He didn't like it when I said this, but he was more like her than he knew."

He did, on occasion, return to something he had stated strongly and attempt to modify its absoluteness, although, on the question of DeSalvo's legal disposition, he never did alter his opinion. Around the time DeSalvo died in prison, my father said, "He *was* in every likelihood the one who carried out all thirteen strangulations. But if the courts were going to convict him, they ought to have done it for the crimes in question—the crimes that they were actually avenging. Instead, they took their vengeance indirectly....

"Anyway, the man should never have been brought to trial."

My father was sixty-one years old at the time DeSalvo wrote that letter to him. He continued with his work for the mental health department and the state judiciary until he was seventy, but he kept on with his practice of psychiatry into his early eighties and never really gave up on the writings he was trying to complete, no matter how chaotic those writings had become, until the year he went into the nursing home.

Twelve more years had passed since then. It was now 2008. My father was 102 years old. In terms of sheer longevity, he had nearly caught up with my mother. But the signs and symptoms of his terminal fragility—"the indications," as he might have worded it—were clear. The final hours of his life, I knew, were near at hand.

CHAPTER TWELVE

The Future in Our Memories

This is how I learned that it was time for me to give up my resistance to finality.

I was in Chicago on a day in August when my father became ill again. He had developed a recurrence of the old infection in his urinary tract and, when Julia notified his doctor, she said she would phone a new prescription to the pharmacy across the street from the apartment. Julia later told me that she felt "a funny kind of hesitation" when she got the medicine and gave the dosage written on the bottle to my father.

"I wasn't sure why I was hesitant at first. Then I spoke to Silvia and I told her what the medicine was called and she said the doctor had prescribed it once about a year before and your father had reacted badly to it." Silvia had been convinced he was allergic to that medicine and, after she had told this to the doctor, she had been instructed not to give him any more.

"I must have had some memory of that under the surface of my mind, but it was too late by then. I'd given him the medicine."

By the end of the afternoon, she said, he was very nauseous and began to vomit. "I didn't wait to call the doctor back. I took him to the hospital."

My plane got into Boston sometime after midnight and, because I had forgotten to turn on my cell phone when the plane had landed, it was not until I walked into my house, an hour north of Boston, that I found a message there from Julia on my answering machine. She had included the name and beeper number of a doctor at the hospital.

The doctor, who responded quickly, reassured me that my father's pulse, although it had been "very low" when he was admitted, was "regular" now and that his temperature was normal. His blood pressure had been high, the doctor said, but had since been stabilized. "I'm confident he'll be okay tonight. If I were you, I'd get some sleep and wait until we have some test results to give you in the afternoon tomorrow."

When I spoke with Julia, who was with my father still and said she would remain there with him at the hospital, she sounded less alarmed than in the message she had left me earlier. "I don't think you should drive all the way back into Boston at this hour. Try to sleep. I'll wake you if there's any change in his condition." The relief in Julia's voice reassured me temporarily. At the same time, I had the premonition that the information I was to be given the next day would not be optimistic.

My father's status remained stable in the morning but, by the early afternoon, I was told he was deteriorating quickly. It was now believed he'd undergone a cardiac arrest before the ambulance had brought him to the hospital. "Blood and oxygen cessation from a cardiac arrest," the senior resident informed me, "does neurological damage. Some of the damage is immediate and some is delayed." Using a term I'd often heard my father use in speaking of brain injury, he explained, "We know that he already underwent a major insult to his brain because of his Alzheimer's. Now he's had a second insult. If he doesn't have another cardiac arrest today, the neurology team will examine him tomorrow to assess his brain-stem functions."

In the "worst-case scenario," he said, "the part of the brain that triggers breathing would no longer function. That's the last thing that the brain gives up. I wish I could tell you...," but I interrupted then to ask how soon my father's life would end if I should determine to take him off his life supports that evening or the next.

"Once we begin the morphine drip, given his condition, it would likely be no more than a few hours."

I told him I would be there before evening.

Efficiency is a convenient anesthetic. I gave myself some time to compile a list of people who would have to be alerted. I sent the list to my assistant. Then I asked her to begin to make "arrangements," which I knew I did not need to specify, because she was prepared for this, but I did it anyway. I tried to reach my sister. I called her several times and left a message on her phone. She traveled often, so I wondered if she was away. I gave my assistant the numbers for my nieces, who, I thought, might reach her before evening. I don't believe she got the message until late at night or early the next morning.

Then I made another list: writings published by my father, dates and markers in his medical career, the years when he began his studies at the MGH and Boston Psychopathic, then at Dr. Meyer's clinic at Johns Hopkins, then when he began his practice in neurology....I did this obsessively. Now I wonder why I wasted time like this instead of simply getting in my car and heading for the hospital. It's possible that making myself very busy in this manner helped me to pretend somehow that things were still as they had been, maybe as they would continue being, even while I knew beyond the slightest doubt that the end of Daddy's life was now at hand.

Possibly, too, I was afraid that if I spent the

hours of the afternoon sitting at his bedside, imagining (as I would surely try to do) that he was giving indications of responsiveness to me or thinking that I could divine some other indications of resilience and vitality, I'd lose the feeling of resolve at which I had arrived. I didn't want to walk into the hospital until I was prepared to let my father die.

Silvia was at his bedside when I came into the room. Julia, who had had no sleep the night before, had finally gone home to rest when Silvia arrived. Silvia had been the most ferocious champion and partisan defender of my father's life as long as any of those satisfactions she religiously detected in him still remained—good appetite, small sparks of humor, spirited resistance to demands she made, or simply that endearing smile, which I sometimes thought was all she asked for in exchange for serving him so faithfully. A single look at Silvia's eyes said everything: acceptance.

The doctor told me that my father's kidneys had shut down. "Most of his other organs have shut down as well. Blood coagulation is no longer functioning." His cerebral condition was now "comatose," the doctor said.

I signed the DNR when it was handed to me. It had no meaning now. An intravenous line was already in his wrist. His face was pale. His eyes were closed. When I bent to kiss him on his cheek, he made not the slightest stir.

The morphine drip began a little after seven. It

was intensified by increments over the next hour and a half. I did not ask Silvia to leave me. Around eight-forty-five, the doctor came back to raise the level slightly. Silvia stepped away from the bed and went to stand beside the window.

From that time on until he died, I held my ear against my father's chest and listened to his breathing as it came at longer, then much longer intervals. At four minutes before nine o'clock, his breathing stopped. The doctor came into the room again, took out his stethoscope, and listened to my father's heart. When he looked up at me, there was nothing that he had to tell me.

My father's doctor showed up in the corridor soon after I had left his room. She came with me and Silvia into a kind of living room at the far end of the floor. Neither Silvia nor I asked her any questions about the medication she'd prescribed to which my father had experienced a bad reaction in the past, but the doctor introduced the subject on her own. "I had no memory," she said, "that your father was allergic to that medicine...." I remember wondering: Didn't doctors take a look at a patient's records when they wrote prescriptions? But I wasn't in a state of mind to pursue the matter.

A few moments later, as I came out to the corridor, where a nurse was waiting to confirm that I had made arrangements for the disposition of my father's body, the young physician with whom I'd developed a close friendship after meeting at my father's bedside when he was in the hospital about three years before came racing from a doorway and, without a single word at first, she put her arms around me and just held me close to her. She told me she had been on duty on another floor but had learned—I didn't ask her how she knew this—that my father had just died. This wonderful, kindhearted doctor, the daughter and granddaughter of physicians as she'd told me, held my hand as she walked me to the elevator bank. When the elevator came, she squeezed my fingers very hard and promised she would call me the next morning.

I got down to the lobby and walked across to the garage and, for the longest time, I couldn't seem to figure out where I'd left my car. Then I walked around one of those concrete posts, up another level, and finally found where I had parked it, and got in and sat there for a while before I turned the engine on. I don't know why I couldn't cry.

Nearly ten years before my father died, while he was in the nursing home, he wrote a memo that contains these words: "We expect more than the common descriptions in popular mockings of penetrating studies. ADVISE: The future remains something in our memories. We are curious, but our patients upon review may benefit.... I look forward to seeing more of you once I am returned to this hemisphere."

In a second memo, he wrote this: "I have recently

been received of a physician who is well spoken of. Materials should be a great help to students—i.e., to totalize and orient the most helpful comments. Soon I may begin to work on these areas of memory of the most serious."

I have had the opportunity to think a great deal since my father's death about the truthfulness of memory. Neuroscience, which has undergone extraordinary breakthroughs over recent years, tells us there are reasons to distrust what we are certain we remember. This is, obviously, not a wholly new idea. Freud, among others in the psychoanalytic schools of the early 1900s, recognized that memory is subject to distortion by unconscious forces that may help us to suppress the pain of past events and allow us to create convincing but fictitious explanations for sufferings we undergo at later stages of our lives. But modern neuroscience carries these ideas considerably further by questioning the very notion that memories exist like so many fixed and hardened entities, "memory deposits" as it were, in some portion of the brain, and that our only challenge, when we remember something, is to extract it, like a bank withdrawal, from the account in which it is contained.

Neuroscientists today would argue that there isn't any bank account, or storage box, in which our memories are waiting for us to retrieve them—to "reach in and pull them out"—but that there is, instead, only the act of remembering itself, in which electrochemical activity between the neurons of the brain re-create portions of a memory that may be accurate reflections of a previous experience but frequently are not.

"Memory is not a literal reproduction of the past," writes Daniel Schacter, the chair of the Department of Psychology at Harvard University and a widely respected scholar of the workings of our memory. It is, instead, "a constructive process" by means of which "bits and pieces of information" that may come from a variety of sources are reassembled, as it were, into a new reality. And that act of reconstruction, he observes, may be affected by a number of distorting factors. One of them, for instance, is the attribution to a past experience of information we possess today but did not have available at the time of the occurrence or the conversation we believe we are remembering. The results of these and other sins of memory, to use Schacter's words, may give us "a skewed rendering of a specific incident"—or, indeed, of more extended episodes of our experience.

Obviously, the notion that we re-create and, in the process, reinvent some portions of our memories runs directly counter to the longing for a sense of certitude that most of us naturally feel about our recollections of people that we loved. Nonetheless, the compelling nature of that argument leads me to reexamine, with perhaps more diligence than otherwise, some of my own memories of my father's life, especially the ones that depend, in turn, on memories that he himself conveyed to me, as well as those my mother has recalled.

Fortunately, many of my memories, and theirs, are corroborated by that plenitude of documents stored here in my home ever since my father shipped them to me, as well as by the others I had found in the apartment that he hadn't had the time to organize.

Among the most delightful of these documents, one that I discovered only recently, is a letter from a woman named Aurélia Thiérrée, the daughter of Victoria Chaplin and a great-granddaughter of Eugene O'Neill, who at the time was living in New York and was soon to embark on what would be a remarkable stage career. According to her letter, she was about to go to work with the film director Milos Forman but was meanwhile working as a volunteer with children in a neighborhood of Harlem. She spoke about the joy she took in tutoring the children but also of her "sense of uselessness" and feelings of "frustration" at how little she could do to alter the conditions of their lives.

Aurélia, as I realized now, had been more than passingly acquainted with my parents. She had come to know them when she had accompanied her mother at some of those times when they entertained Victoria in Boston. "Our dinners together remain," she wrote, "some of the most agreeable and fascinating memories I keep. Hearing from you about my great-grandfather was priceless in its depth of meaning to me. Thank you!"

I had sometimes wondered if the intimacy of my parents' friendship with the Chaplins and their children had been overstated in my mother's recollections. Now I was happy to discover, in Aurélia's beautifully handwritten letter, that the many stories my mother had told Julia about her closeness to Aurélia's family had not merely been the sweet concoctions of the years when she began to entertain herself with fantasies.

Letters from Oona, of which I have read several—affectionate and impulsive letters and, until her husband's death, generally cheerful, filled with news about her children—have a similar effect in countering whatever doubts I may have had about my mother's memory. ("Geraldine just had a baby boy," she wrote in 1974, "and is on top of the world....The rest of the family [is] keeping out of jail, so life is very pleasant....")

Other letters that I've read from relatives of people Daddy treated represent a different kind of affirmation—reinforcing, for example, memories that I'd retained about his methods of examination and the way that he negotiated complicated family situations. Then, too, there is the information I have now and then received in person as the consequence of a chance encounter with a man or woman who was once in treatment with him.

Two months after Daddy's death, I was at a university in Pennsylvania to make a presentation to the undergraduates. At the end of my talk, a woman who appeared to be in her early fifties, or maybe slightly older, introduced herself to me and, after telling me about her work with troubled and disabled children, said, "I knew your father. He was my doctor when I was a teenage girl. I'd love to talk with you someday and share some of my memories."

The two of us soon began a correspondence. The story she told me of the treatment she was given by my father reminded me of several of his other cases in that she was not the only member of her family he had treated. "You see," she said, "before I knew your father, he had helped my father when he underwent a serious depression. At the same time, he was giving counsel to my mother because she had to bear the burden of my father's illness. So he was seeing both of them at once, helping my father to emerge from his depression while giving my mother emotional support to keep her on an even keel while she was coping with my father."

Her father, she said, had been an active man, but, when he was nearly fifty, he had had an orthopedic problem that temporarily prevented him from walking, and it had been handled badly by an orthopedic specialist, who told him that the problem in all likelihood was irreversible and that he would probably be in a wheelchair soon. "That was when he fell into this terrible depression. He couldn't continue with his work. Before long, he'd withdrawn from almost everything outside our home, until it occurred to him or to my mother to reach out to your father, who had been a friend of his in college....

"I don't know exactly what your father did, but my mother said he was incensed by the behavior of the orthopedic specialist. I think he brought him to another doctor, another specialist, somebody he trusted. His own treatment of my father was purely psychiatric, to get him out of that depression, and it was amazingly successful. My father was walking normally again within another year. Thanks to God, there was never any wheelchair!"

About ten years had passed, she said, before she had to face a crisis of her own. "I was eighteen at the time and I wanted to drop out of college. That's not so unusual these days but, when I was growing up, 'good girls' didn't do that. And I had been a 'good girl' and had always tried to do exactly what my parents had expected. But suddenly I realized I wasn't ready yet to be in college. I didn't want to be there. I was feeling panicky and underwent anxiety attacks. I worried how my parents would react to this....

"When I told the college that I wanted to take off a year, they said I'd need to get a medical excuse for leaving if I ever wanted to return. The college sent me to its own psychiatrist, some doctor that the college had retained, I guess, to deal with problems like this. I hated him! I refused to talk with him.

239

"So, finally, I called my parents and my father said, 'I have this friend in Boston....' So he sent me to your father. And I'm fairly sure my father hoped that he would calm me down, help me to restore my sense of confidence, and send me back to college. This is what I loved about your father: He said that it made perfect sense for me to take a year from college, since I didn't have the least idea why I was there! He told me there was nothing wrong with my decision and I didn't need to be afraid that it would have some dreadful consequence. Once I had a chance to gain a little more experience in life, maybe find an interesting job, or go abroad or to some other section of the country and perhaps just 'look around at things' without the feeling that I had a sword above my head, he was confident I'd recognize the time when I was ready to go back to school. He also said he would predict, in spite of all the bluster that the college had put up, they'd probably be glad to have me back.

"This is the thing: He was empowering to me. There was no sense of dire warnings and no sense of issuing commands. He never made me helplessly dependent, but he enabled me to learn enough about myself so that I could grow into a strong young woman who was capable of making my own judgments. He had this way of personalizing everything he said to me and, once I had made up my mind, he fought for me fiercely....

"At the same time he understood how much I

loved my father and he knew I didn't want to hurt him. He handled this so carefully! I mean: the way he could delineate between the suffering that I was going through, and the decision I had made, and the vulnerability to which this might expose my father. I feel so blessed that he was able to bring out the best in both of us and leave us feeling closer to each other."

Ultimately, she told me, "when I was ready, I returned to college." She went on to study law, then grew attracted to the problems faced by young adults and children and, after marrying happily and having children of her own, proceeded to carve out a new career as a special education advocate, in which, she says, she's found a great deal of fulfillment.

"What I remember best about your father was this truly rare ability he had to transcend the boundary between his friendship with my family and his determination to enable me to reach the very core of who I was and what I needed to feel safe and whole. He was uniquely able to maintain the professional distance necessary to protect his role as my psychiatrist while at the same time acting as my trusted friend. In my work with children and their parents, I always try to keep in mind the model that he set for me. I thank him to this day for the gift he gave me."

After I'd been corresponding with this woman for a while, I got to know her better when she came to Boston for Thanksgiving and invited me to spend an evening with her mother, who, at the age of eighty-five, still remembered vividly how furious my father was with the orthopedic specialist who told her husband he would never walk again. She also had a nice nostalgic memory of going fishing with my father and her husband some years later and my father's great delight in pulling out a pickerel from a river near their home. I was reminded of the tackle box and those rods and marbled reels that were still in my garage....

A sensible awareness of the way that memory may frequently mislead us notwithstanding, memories recorded by so many different people and those that are preserved in so many of the notes and other documents my father left behind tend to reinforce each other. For good or ill, he left so large a volume of materials that even now I have yet to make my way through more than half these packages and file cases and have scrutinized only a small portion of the items they contain. Will I ever have the opportunity to look at all the rest? If he were alive to counsel me, I suspect he'd recommend that I should leave it to a person of a younger generation, perhaps a medical historian, maybe an archivist of modern neuroscience as it was evolving in my father's day, to look at those materials for whatever value they may hold.

I think my father, in all likelihood, would tell me that I should no longer dwell upon remainders and reminders of a life lived largely in a century that's passed. "Get on with your own work now. You have better things to do than try to make sense of another man's existence." That sounds like something he might say to me, or to a patient, in a moment of frustration with obsessive efforts to recapture every detail of the works and days that others, even those we loved, have now completed.

Still, every time I go up to the attic of my house, where all those documents are stored, I feel the strongest inclination to open up another set of folders and see what they may hold. Not long ago, I pulled out a transcript of my father's grades from Harvard College in his freshman year. He got honors grades in English and philosophy, and a C in history, but I was surprised to find that he received a D in his first semester of psychology. He somehow brought it up to an A in the next semester. That was in the spring of 1924. I don't know why I find myself attracted to these unimportant details. I guess I'm not quite ready yet to give in to finality.

Epilogue: 2015

I began these memoirs in September of 2008, a month after my father died. I continued writing through the winter of that year and the spring that followed. I finished in the summer of 2009.

At that point, I set aside these pages and continued with my work, visiting in public schools, interviewing teachers, lecturing at colleges, and writing about inner-city children, as I'd done for most of my career. In this way, I kept myself preoccupied as the aftermath of mourning dwindled down. It was a long time after that before I was ready to open up this manuscript again.

Today, as I read this story of my parents' lives and the way that I remembered them after they had died, there's not a great deal I would change, but, with the distance time affords, there are some important things that I would add.

After losing both my parents in so short a time, and with my father's final year so keenly in my mind, I couldn't bring myself to dwell at any length on moments when a thread of tension drifted through our lives. I mentioned once that I sometimes hurt my father unintendingly and that he sometimes caused me pain as well; but I added nothing more—I didn't want to think of it.

The truth is that not every bit of tension that came up between us was quite as slight or evanescent as I have implied. There were areas of disagreement—most of them about the course of my career—that could be, on some occasions, almost confrontational. At these times, I felt disarmed to a degree by the commanding and authoritative role he had always held for me.

The power that he exercised over my state of mind was magnified, I'm sure, by my early recognition of the power that he wielded over other people's lives. I recall, for instance, that when I was eight or nine he brought me with him to the MGH to observe a neurosurgical procedure that one of his colleagues was performing on a patient whom my father had been treating. I have a memory of standing there beside him on some kind of balcony, just above the operating area, as he was communicating with the surgeon while the surgeon was removing a brain tumor from his patient.

My father and the surgeon were talking with each other by the use of tiny microphones. (The area where we were standing was divided from the operating theater by a glass partition.) The knowledge that my father's judgment and the guidance he appeared to be providing to the surgeon might, in part, determine if his patient would emerge from the procedure with his faculties intact did not leave me simply with the sense of fascination any child, I imagine, would have taken from that neurosurgical arena. It was more like an enduring imprint of amazement that so much seemed to be resting on my father's intuition and interpretation of the E.E.G. his patient had been given, as well as on the careful and decisive motions of those white-gloved fingers just beneath us. Only someone godlike was, I thought, supposed to have this kind of power.

I have no idea if my father could have guessed the full effect that this would have on me. I do know this experience and others like it in the years to come left me with a sense of awe and admiration for my father that would render me more eager than a child probably should ever be to look for his approval as I got into my teenage years and then went on to college. His approval, I would soon discover, wasn't going to be given easily.

At the end of my freshman year at Harvard, for example, when students were ranked numerically according to their grades, my roommate's ranking was among the highest in our class. My own grades were also good, but they were lower than my room-mate's. As comical as it may seem to anyone except for me, my father made a comment, the words of which I've managed to forget, that gave me the distinct impression that I'd disappointed him. Like many Harvard students, I had been ranked at the head of my class while I was in secondary school. My father expected I would keep on in this pattern at the university. For a man who chastised many of the parents of his patients for holding their own children to unrealistic and unhealthy expectations, my father's uncontrollable competitiveness on my behalf seemed almost inexplicable.

By my junior year, when I began two years of study with the poet Archibald MacLeish, I was able for the most part to dismiss my father's pressures, for which I'm grateful to MacLeish, who told me, when I wrote a piece for him (which I unconvincingly disguised as "fiction") about a father who was over-bearingly ambitious for his son, that I should "take it easy" and allow myself to have some fun while I was in college. He even spurred me on when he detected my infatuation with one of the two Radcliffe students in our class.

Still, I continued to study hard and in the spring of junior year I was one of the eight members of my class who were elected, one year early, to Phi Beta Kappa. At a dinner that was held in order to induct us into PBK, we were required to elect one of our fellow members to serve as the "first marshal" of our class at our graduation a year later. One of my friends, Jared Diamond, whom I'd known since we were in secondary school, was sitting near me at the table. Jared was not only, as I thought, by far the smartest boy I'd ever known; he also had a lovely sense of humor and (as he still does) a likable and self-effacing personality. I thought he ought to be the one to represent us.

My father, whom I had invited to the dinner, looked disappointed when I nominated Jared. I don't recall if Jared won or if it was another member of our group who was chosen as first marshal. But I do remember that my father was unhappy. At the end of dinner, as I walked him to his car, he said to me, "All the same, it would have made me proud if it was you who was selected." I remember standing with him on a corner of Mount Auburn Street, a block from Harvard Square, as he unlocked his car, still looking discontent. As I watched him driving off, I was sorry I'd invited him.

My father's high ambitions for me were appeased, but only briefly, when, in my final year of college, I was awarded a Rhodes Scholarship to Oxford. (It was, I've always been convinced, MacLeish's strong and generous endorsement that led to my selection.) As it turned out, however, I was bored by the curriculum at Oxford and greatly disappointed when the tutor I had been assigned told me she did not allow her students to concentrate on modern British authors—which, of course, prohibited my wish to write my thesis on a living poet, W. H. Auden, and on the Irish poet William Butler Yeats. Then, too, the atmosphere among the undergraduates and graduates I got to know struck me as more socially class-conscious, and uncomfortably so, than what I had experienced at Harvard.

I went to Paris for the winter break and, encouraged by some older writers I encountered—William Styron was in Paris at the time, as was his friend and fellow novelist James Jones—I decided to remain there. I showed the writing I was doing to my newfound mentors and, with their help, sold one of my stories to a European magazine. With these meager earnings and the royalties from a piece of juvenilia I had published in the fall, I was just barely able to support myself.

MacLeish, after having helped me to receive my scholarship to Oxford, was not in the least disturbed by my decision to abandon it. My father, on the other hand, told me I was making "an egregious mistake." He wrote me some horrendously alarming letters, in which he said he hoped I would return to England promptly and continue with my scholarship—"before you find that it's too late."

The encouragement he'd given other people of my age not to be afraid to interrupt their studies and go out into the world and look around a little, and to defend their need for independence without fear of repercussions, whatever they might be, as he'd conveyed this to one of the patients I've described, was not to be replicated in the case of his own son. When, in a defensive letter, I reminded him of his decision to give up Harvard Law School and the time of wandering and searching for direction he'd allowed himself, not only then but even after he'd become a doctor, he replied that he was "amused" but "not convinced" by my attempt to claim his own experience as precedent.

"I wasn't a Rhodes Scholar," he said bluntly. "This is a different ballpark altogether. I don't think you understand the risks that you're incurring." He said that my decision troubled him "considerably."

After I returned to Boston, he was mightily relieved when I told him I was thinking of going back to Harvard to pursue a doctorate under the guidance of my former teachers. But his anxieties came to the fore again when, in the rising turmoil of the civil rights campaigns, I abruptly changed my mind and, as I have noted, decided to become a teacher at an elementary school in the black community of Roxbury. My father didn't openly oppose this but he told my mother he was worried by the seeming randomness and suddenness of my decision.

He would later reconsider his objections as it grew apparent to him that I had at last arrived at something he regarded as at least a temporary desti- nation. And when, in the years ahead, he recognized that it wasn't going to be temporary and when, unex- pectedly, it led me back to writing and, at last, to publication of a book about the children I was teaching that he genuinely admired, his concerns about me seemed to be allayed.

I was fortunate that a social critic and psychiatrist named Robert Coles, whom my father held in high esteem, gave the book a good review in the New York Times. My father told me that he found this "gratifying." And when, in the spring that followed, I was given a National Book Award, he took me to dinner at the Harvard Club, the two of us alone, and said that, "all in all," he was "very pleased." He even conceded that he now believed he had been in error in the reservations he had had when I became a teacher.

Nonetheless, I can't forget the look of grimness and foreboding in his eyes when I first ventured into Roxbury. Even though he had restrained himself from telling me, as he told my mother, that he feared I'd "lost [my] bearings" and that I was going to regret the choices I was making, the admonitory undertone I heard within his voice in almost every conversation that we had that year was not easy to dismiss.

As late as five years after that, in the early 1970s, I discovered that I still was not exempt from the power that my father wielded over me. This was at a time when the civil rights campaigns to which I had attached myself were starting to disintegrate after having lost their most dynamic leaders either to assassination or to the attrition of their stamina as they were growing older, while others were the casualties of self-destructive personal behavior. My father, who could read my mind with the same acuity he brought into his work as a clinician, was able to detect the mild stirrings of uneasiness I underwent as I watched increasing numbers of the activists and younger leaders I had known, especially the ones whose motivations had been rooted in their ideologies, abandoning the causes to which they'd been committed since their days as undergraduates.

My own beliefs remained unchanged. I had not become involved in civil rights out of ideology but out of the sense that, if I stepped back from the fray, I would be avoiding an obligation that belonged to people of my age at that moment in our history— a feeling that was deepened by the visceral experience of teaching my young students and observing the conditions of immiseration in the neighborhood in which they lived. So the rapidly changing ideological environment and the splintering of left-wing groups had little effect upon the work that I was doing or the books that I was writing. Nonetheless, it was increasingly apparent that the activist mentality of many of the students I'd been meeting at the universities was rapidly diminishing. In part because there was no longer any movement to sustain and mobilize their idealistic energies, they seemed to see no concrete ways to act on their beliefs. With this, inevitably, there was a fading of audacity: a loss of urgency and fervor.

Within another year or two, my father recognized that I was starting to experience more than a "mild stirring" of uneasiness about the changes taking place around me, but he also realized that I was unable or unwilling to adapt to these political realities. I think he decided I could use a wake-up call. When he sat down with me one evening in his home, he got directly to the point.

"I've been watching you the past few years," he said, "and, if you want to know what I've been thinking, I won't sugarcoat it for you. Here's what I believe. You're still living as if you regard yourself as some kind of mild-mannered, Harvard-educated reembodiment of Che Guevara. But your soldiers in blue jeans are going back to business school. They're thinking about salaries and mortgage payments, not about a revolution....I think I know you better than you know yourself. I'm your father. I want to see you thinking hard about what I've just said to you."

His choice of words ("soldiers in blue jeans") startled me, to say the least. I was anything but a revolutionary by the standards of the times. But I think the gravity of his concern was heightened by the fact that a number of the few remaining activists I knew had been attracted, since the last years of the 1960s, into some alarmingly irrational and violent activities. The emergence of a group known as the Weather Underground had been given wide attention in the press. As a psychiatrist, my father was convinced that they were living in a world of fantasy—"total detachment," as he put it, "from the slightest recognition of the damage that they're doing to the very causes they claim to believe in."

He said he'd been relieved when I openly discredited this group and others like it. But I think he worried nonetheless that I was at risk of being drawn, not into destructive or irrational activities, but into incendiary writings that would marginalize me in a manner that would undermine my possible effectiveness and also (I am sure that this was in his mind) might endanger my ability to earn a living as an author.

If my father had not been so knowledgeable about the ways that people, at destabilizing moments in their lives, often fall into behavior that intensifies their instability, I might have found it easier to write off his anxieties, as I'd done before. But this time I think I knew my father was correct. In subsequent years, I found that I was grateful for the sobering effect his good advice had had. I think it helped me understand my situation more realistically.

In the early 1980s, after Ronald Reagan became president and the shift in the political terrain that had begun during the Nixon years was crystallized in the revanchist policies not only of severe conservatives but also of some very smart and bitter former radicals and liberals who seemed to look with horror at their earlier ideals and with contempt for those who still adhered to them, I underwent a second crisis of self-questioning. Once again, I spoke about this with my father. This time, it was I who opened up the conversation.

At some point in 1983, I had brought a book proposal to my literary agent that described a work I had begun about the many adults I was meeting, most of them in very poor communities, who could barely read, if they could read at all, and therefore couldn't help their children in their preschool years or when they entered public school. I had started working with some literacy groups and had written a preliminary paper, a battle plan of sorts, for programs that would be designed to teach these parents and their children simultaneously—a plan that was adopted by the California system of state libraries. The book that I proposed would build upon this work, but carry it much further.

My agent, however, recognizing that this project, because of its inner-city emphasis, represented a continuation of my writings about race and the effects of systematic inequality, told me that he didn't think there would be much interest from a publisher. "Times have changed. The readership for books like this is disappearing quickly. If I were you, I'd start to think of moving on to something new."

I was stunned when he rejected my proposal. But his statement—"times have changed"—left me with the fear that he might have a better sense than I of what the market possibilities were like. I became so shaken in my confidence that I worked myself into a state of mind in which I worried that the books I had already published might be going out of print and heading for remainder bins.

By this date, many of my leftist friends who could see the way the pendulum was swinging were trying to secure positions in the academic world, typically at universities or colleges of a progressive bent. When I spoke about this with my father, his first reaction was to say that this "might not be such a bad idea" for me to think about as well.

I think he knew that I'd been given academic invitations in the past and had rather blithely turned them down. But not long after we had had that conversation, I received an inquiry that held some real appeal for me. It was a position in a subject area that crossed department boundaries—"social ethics," "social justice," something of that sort—at one of the more exclusive academic institutions in New England. The invitation followed soon after a lecture I had given there; and in my first burst of relief, and expecting that my father would be pleased, I drove directly into Boston to regale him with this news.

By the time I got to the apartment, however, and started to describe this to my father, I had begun to think about it with conflicted feelings. On the one hand, the invitation had been tendered to me by a socially committed man who, I knew, was not expecting me, and did not want me, to submit to any cooling down of my beliefs, which, at first sight, I had thought the social milieu in which I'd be working might require. "This old institution could use some shaking up," he said. "To be quite honest, I think you could help me...."

On the other hand, because I'd visited classes like the ones that I presumably would teach, I told my father that I wasn't wholly comfortable with the idea of spending the next twenty years of my career teaching very fortunate young people instead of working, as I'd done in the preceding years, with kids who never had these opportunities.

My father held back from reacting for a while. His hands were clasped. He was looking at me thoughtfully. I reminded him of one of the kids I'd taught in Roxbury, whom I knew he would remember, a terribly unhappy boy named Stephen who mumbled to himself in class and was routinely beaten with a bamboo whip, after it was dipped in vinegar, which was an accepted form of discipline in the city's "negro schools" in 1965. He grew into his teenage years with a sense of rage and vengefulness and my father tried to intervene on his behalf after he committed an atrocious crime that led to his imprisonment.

I told my father that I didn't like the thought of marching out a little boy like Stephen, and the many other inner-city children I had come to know, as if they were so many social specimens to touch the edges of the conscience of those who were more privileged than they and whose advantages, at least to some degree, depended on the inequalities I'd seen.

It was true, of course, that I had written about Stephen and his classmates and others in his neighborhood, but I was also living in the black community, and working among families there, and I thought my writing was affected by that vantage point. Living and teaching in an affluent environment would be a major change in course for me. I said I was convinced that others with experience akin to mine could cross that line between the two extremes in our society with loyalties intact and do it in a graceful way that would not compromise their feelings of integrity. But I wasn't sure that I could make that crossing—or whether it would be a good idea for me even to try.

This was one of the moments for which I'll always be most grateful to my father. He had listened to me patiently. But when he spoke at last, he utterly surprised me.

"Don't do it!" he said. "It's not for you. I've had a chance to think about this since you talked about those friends of yours looking for positions in the academic world." He told me that he now regretted the hasty way he had reacted at the time. The invitation I'd described to him was "flattering," he said, and he could see why it initially appealed to me. But he added that he found my second thoughts about it more in keeping with his own.

"It would, in a sense, be 'cashing in your chips.' I don't think you'll be at peace if you agree to do this."

He said that, since our earlier talk, he had discussed the issue of my publication worries and my possible return to academia with my mother and that I should talk about this with her if I wanted and I'd find that she agreed with him. "We don't think you need to run for safety. We think you'll survive these next few years just fine." Even with Mr. Reagan in the White House, he went on, "there's got to be a vast number of people who rebel against the shallowness and meanness of his policies. Every decent instinct in this nation didn't die when he came into office." And, he said, no matter what my agent told me, he was convinced that there were many publishers who would take an interest in the book I had in mind. "I'm also certain that you'll find your readers are still there—maybe scattered, maybe very quiet now, maybe somewhat hidden in the crevices.... I'm confident that they're still there."

He got up from his chair. He'd been sitting at his desk but now he walked across the room and took an ashtray from the sideboard in the dining area. I believe I've mentioned that my father liked to smoke a pipe. On the sideboard there was a leather-covered humidor. He packed his pipe and lighted it.

"The very nice position you described would be a throwback for you. Something in you turned against that kind of life when you gave up your Rhodes and decided to leave Oxford, and you know I was unhappy with you at the time. I wanted to fly over there and drag you back, but your mother wouldn't let me. I didn't think you knew what you were doing. Or, if you did, I didn't think you could sustain it. I was wrong...."

Standing near one of the windows as he drew upon his pipe, the smoke from the expensive blend he liked drifting up about him, and gazing out across the river at the skyline of the universities on the Cambridge side, he allowed himself another pause before he spoke again.

"I don't think I've ever said this to you in so many words, but I'm glad you went the way you did. And now, after you've staked so much, I don't want to see you turning back. I want you to keep on."

At the door when I was putting on my coat, he said again, with all the old authority his voice commanded for me still, "You're going to be fine!" He tapped me on the shoulder then. "By the way, get rid of that agent if you can. It doesn't sound as if he's been much of a friend to you."

I followed his advice. A few weeks later, I telephoned a better and far more respected agent, named Lynn Nesbit, who has been my agent ever since. A month later, she sent me a contract for the book I had proposed. When it was published, in 1985, it reached a good-size audience and, I'd like to think, helped to bring attention to the needs of men and women whose shabby education, or lack of education, had denied them the ability to read. It also earned enough to keep me going for two years. Then I settled down once more into the writing of those books about our children and their schools that matter most to me.

Less than seven years went by between the night my father gave me that advice and the time when he began to lose his line of thought in the course of conversation and started having trouble with his memory of people's names or the names of places he was trying to describe. Before long, there was also a perceptible decline in his sense of confidence about decisions he was making for my mother and himself.

From that point on, the balance of power between us started shifting. Now it was he who began to ask for my suggestions on occasion and to look to me for reassurance when he fell into uncertainties about the papers he was writing—even though the pieces he was showing me continued to be skillfully developed, and some of them, I thought, were strikingly original. He wasn't simply reconfiguring arguments he'd made and conclusions he'd arrived at in the past, as thoughtful people, intellectuals and others, often tend to do when they get into later years. Indeed, in several of these pieces, there was an unquestioned evolution in his thinking and a new emboldenment in giving voice to points of view that were more provocative than anything he'd written up to now.

One of the most compelling of these papers was an effort to refine positions he had taken earlier in his career on ethical considerations to be brought to bear, on the part of a psychiatrist, in evaluation of a dissident behavior that might be regarded by conventional opinion as an unacceptable offense to civic order. In the beginning of the paper, he drew a sharp distinction between pathological behavior or irrational destructiveness and what he termed "a principled resistance" to societal injustice. "Rage at oppression," he observed, "has been considered righteous from time immemorial." Even actions of explicit violence, he said, have been "tolerated, even welcomed," when "the absence of alternatives has engendered desperation...."

He went on to say that he did not equate criminally dangerous behavior "with contemporary patterns of societal remonstrance" in the United States or elsewhere, "although the remonstrants may be perceived as dangerous by targeted establishments." He spoke respectfully of those whose motivation "is essentially altruistic (based on compassionate identification with others)," as opposed to those whose motivation must be seen as "egoistic" and originating from unhealthy rage in a disordered personality. The empathetic way in which he spoke of "principled resistance" struck me, when I read this, not as a rejection of his earlier beliefs but certainly as a rather daring emendation of anything I'd known him to express before.

A week or so after he had shown this paper to me, he sent me a photocopy of a piece of writing by an Italian philosopher of the eighteenth century, with a commentary written by Voltaire, entitled "Crimes and Punishments," which he had found at the medical school, where he had been spending many hours in the famous Countway Library while he'd been working on his paper. He said it wasn't relevant to the points that he was making, but he'd marked a passage that he thought I'd find of interest.

The passage began, "Finally, the most certain method of preventing crimes is to perfect the system of education. But this is...an object, if I may venture to declare it, which is so intimately connected with the nature of government that it will always remain a barren spot...." My father said, "I thought perhaps you might like to quote this in one of your lectures." He had circled the words "will always remain a barren spot." This enjoyable collegiality between us would continue for a while longer.

Within another year, however, I was forced to recognize a heightened sense of insecurity, reflected, for example, in the disproportionate degree of gratitude he would express for the small amounts of help I had been giving him. I had begun to do my best to mediate between him and my mother as their tensions with each other were increasing. I was also doing what I could to help him keep his notes and papers organized. I noticed that his desk was cluttered with a lot of semi-finished pages and suggested that he paper-clip related items and sequence them thematically, so he wouldn't feel so overwhelmed when he went back to writing the next morning.

"Dear Jonathan," he wrote to me soon after that, "your visit has done more for me and mother than only you can know. Your directness [this was in reference to his quarrels with my mother] and your good suggestion that I organize my workplace and clean up the mess you noticed on my desk encouraged me to make a start at this, and I did, and have already made considerable progress. I am encouraged. I shall go on with this and keep you informed...."

But that feeling of encouragement was obviously fragile. In the fall of 1991, when he was invited to address a convocation on terrorist activities, which was to take place in Rome in the first week of December, his growing recognition of the failings of his memory led him into several weeks of painful indecision.

"My anxiety is dreadful," he reported in a letter that he sent me in October. I notice now that, on the envelope, he had placed twice the number of postage stamps needed for so short a letter and had written my address in very large block letters with my street and zip code underlined with a thick black marker.

The letter makes it evident that he had gone into a tailspin of self-doubt about the lecture he would be presenting at this convocation, at which, he knew, a number of his European colleagues would be present. As soon as I read this, I got on the phone and asked if he would like to let me see a copy of the paper. When he said he thought that it might give him some perspective if we could sit down and read it through together, I got in my car and headed down to Boston. He had the paper waiting for me in the living room when I arrived.

The paper focused on the psychiatric disposition of an individual who was prepared to put his life at risk, and perhaps the lives of others, by participating in an act of violence—the hijack of an aircraft, for example—in pursuit of a political agenda. "Acts of antisocial violence," he had begun, "frequently involve an identificational blurring between the self and others, the aggressor and his victims." In such acts, as he surmised, "the aggressor's behavior appears to have a wraithlike quality of self-immolation." He expanded on his reference to "self-immolation" by hypothesizing that this might at times take on "a self-enhancing quality" or "some kind of theological dimension."

Again, as in the previous paper he had shown me, he distinguished such behavior from those acts of violence that might be regarded from some points of view as rational responses to oppressive situations. And while he made it more than clear that he was not condoning terrorist activities, he gave a nuanced recognition of the fact that violent behavior cannot always be perceived as pathological and that historians—"as in the instance," he suggested, "of the slave revolts in the United States"—have frequently regarded such behavior as courageous and heroic, even though this point of view is almost always angrily contested.

When I finished reading this, I told my father right away that I thought it was terrific. If only for the line about "a wraithlike quality of self-immolation," I said that I was certain the conferees in Rome would find this of great interest. At his request, I marked some repetitions, added three or four transitions, and suggested some resequencing of passages.

Six weeks after that, he flew to Italy with my mother for the convocation. If he had to struggle now and then with lapses in his memory—and I assume he did—I imagine that he managed to glide over them or otherwise disguise them with his usual agility. On the basis of notations that he made after his presentation, the reaction from the other conferees left him with the sense of satisfaction he had hoped for and I had expected.

After the conference, he and my mother extended their stay, the last such trip they'd ever make, by traveling to Florence and Assisi. Then, as a special treat to celebrate my mother's birthday—she was eighty-eight on the fifteenth of the month—they went on to Venice, which they'd never visited before,

and spent part of a week there with one of his colleagues from Toronto and a young Italian doctor they
had met in Rome.

A tender note he'd written to my mother on the
stationery of the Gritti Palace, the hotel in which they
stayed in Venice, gave me the impression that the
extra weeks in Italy had been my father's late-in-life
attempt to make amends, as insufficient as I'm sure
he knew they were, for the many times of grief and
worry he had caused her in their years of marriage.
"I want you to know that I have always loved you
and am grateful for the patience you have shown me.
It was you who recognized my hunger to become a
doctor at a time when others had discouraged me. I
am so thankful for the many years in which you have
guided me and cared for me...."

Even then, however, while they were in Venice,
my father's usual congenial manner and quick-witted
gift for making friends with strangers had, it seems,
brought him the attention of an attractive woman
who was seated near him at a dinner party, given
in his honor as I gathered, and my mother seems to
have decided that he had been too responsive to the
woman's interest.

"At your age, Harry," she had written to him
after they came home, in one of the many letters they
would leave for one another in the kitchen, propped
against the coffeepot, "you should be ashamed to
pay attention to that kind of woman." Using an old-
fashioned word, my mother had described the

woman as "some kind of floozy." The matter, bless-edly, ended there. My father naturally told my mother he was sorry he had hurt her feelings.

Six months after their return to Boston, my father sat me down for the conversation, the one he tape-recorded, in which he described to me the epi-sodes of "cutoff"—"interrupted consciousness"—he had started to experience, and their probable causation. It was another eighteen months before he had the consultation with his former student that confirmed the diagnosis.

Two years after that, his primary physician, who had been a friend of his for more than thirty years, wrote to his attorney, "Harry has become incapable of managing his own affairs by reason of advanced age and mental incapacity." By June of that year, fol-lowing his accident, he was in the nursing home. The tilting of the balance between my father's exercise of competence and judgment and authority in help-ing me get through some of the most uncertain and unstable times in my career and my own responsi-bility to count upon my competence and judgment to protect him in the years that now remained had come to be essentially complete.

From that time on, whenever any memories of early disagreements or ancient-seeming tensions between my father and myself drifted back into my mind, I did my best to banish them in their totality. Instead, I gravitated to the best of memories. I'd find myself drawn back consolingly to early mornings on the lake in Maine when the fish were biting or, as we were always able to persuade ourselves when we saw a ripple on the surface of the water, curiously nibbling. I'd also recollect the times he brought me with him when he was rushing off to see a patient in the evening, and I'd open up his doctor's bag again and hold the tuning fork or wooden throat sticks in my hand. Or I would remember (maybe my favorite memory of all) his putting the stethoscope around my neck and lifting me onto a patient's bed, letting me pretend I was his "chief assistant." Pride in my father, thankfulness that he had been my father, and an ultimately grateful feeling of respect (grudging at first, it took a while to come) for the aching if imperfect love he never ceased to feel for Mom—these are the things I wanted to hold on to.

It will soon be seven years since the night I bent down by his bed to press my ear against his chest and listen to his breathing as his life came to its end. But even now, and even after rounding out the story of his sometimes turbulent complexity, as I've felt obliged to do in order to keep faith with the reality of who he was, it is the reaffirming memories that crowd out all the rest.

The sense that I was on a journey with my father—seventy-two years is a good big piece of anybody's life—did not end abruptly on the day I buried him. On cold November nights when I'm in a thoughtful mood or worried about problems with my work, or personal missteps I may have made, and go out walking by myself along the country roads around my house, I like to imagine that he's there beside me still, tapping that old cane of his, making his amusing comments on the unpredictable events and unexpected twists and turns in other people's lives.

Perhaps, over the next few years, that sense of his continuing companionship will fade. It probably will. But some part of the legacy my father and good mother gave me will, I know, remain with me even when their voices and their words and the expressions on their faces and the vivid details of their life's adventure become attenuated in the course of time. Some of the blessings that our parents give us, I need to believe, outlive the death of memory.

ACKNOWLEDGMENTS

A great many kind and patient people have helped me in the writing of this book and given me encouragement to bring it to completion. I thank especially Caroline Jalfin, Cassie Schwerner, Amy Ehntholt, Melanie Harris, Julia Barnard, Jacey Rubinstein, Daniel O'Leary, Dr. Lisa Rosenbaum, Jane Dimyan-Ehrenfeld, Ariella Suchow, and my editors Domenica Alioto and Doug Pepper. Thanks, too, to Dr. Edward Rabe, Dr. Jim Roseto, Dr. Emily Coskun, Dr. Michael Johnson, and Dr. Lawrence Hartmann, who reviewed portions of this book and helped me to correct or clarify references to medical and neuropsychiatric probems and procedures.

My deepest debt is to my close friends and assistants Vanessa Krasinski and Lily Jones. Lily did the lion's share of the research on this book, helped me to sort out hundreds of my father's papers, and tried to check my father's memories against whatever published documents were available. Vanessa worked painstakingly on almost every aspect of the book in its final stages. I thank them both for their persistence.

I'm grateful also to Aurélia Thiérrée, a great-granddaughter of Eugene O'Neill and a gifted stage-performer, who read this book as I was working on the first twelve chapters, told me of her meetings with my parents and later, when we spent some time together, helped me to confirm my mother's recollections of her family.

Some of the people who brought the greatest comfort to my parents in their later years—Julia Walker, Silvia Garcia, Angela and Alejandro Gomez, and the nurse I call Lucinda—have been described at length. But there were others, of whom I haven't spoken or have done so only passingly.

One of them was Linda Hiller, the daughter of my father's younger brother, whose emotional support and kindness to my father never wavered in his final years. Another was Michael Meyer, a teaching assistant at the University of Massachusetts, who became immersed in my father's writings, sometimes helped him to do research, and frequently stayed overnight at the apartment to calm the tensions that arose between him and my mother. Yet another was the loyal student from Nepal who drove in from Amherst to keep my father company while he was in the nursing home and, like Alejandro, had a special gift for making intellectual connections with my father. He soon became a part of that inner circle of good friends and helpers who brought a sense of continuity and warm familiarity into my father's life. I wish I'd had a chance to speak of all these people in more detail.

I've also spoken only briefly of my sister. This is

largely the result of geographic distance. She didn't live here—as I've noted, she had moved to the Midwest more than forty years before—and therefore didn't have the opportunity to be present in the day-to-day events and observe the slowly changing rhythms in our parents' lives or take an active role in the decision-making that was needed, almost always at short notice. But another reason is the very narrow scope and focus of this book. One of the imperfections in the way I've told this story is a kind of tunnel vision, or partially closed lens, that arrows in upon those aspects of my father's life and mine that we shared with one another, to the relative exclusion of other aspects of his life, no matter how important, that remain on the periphery.

I've described the feeling that I often had of traveling at my father's side as if I were alone with him for extended periods of time—a feeling that intensified when he sat me down and described to me, in confidence, the early indications of his sickness and later as we struggled to make sense out of his puzzlements and uncompleted sentences and increasingly fragmented memories.

In reality, we were not alone. Until a year before her death, my mother was there, close at hand, strong of will, and for the most part clear of mind. My sister came to Boston at least twice a year, and often more, to spend time at the nursing home and visit the apartment. Her children, both of whom had settled in New England, came to Boston frequently.

Her older daughter, Jody, who lived in Massachusetts and had a deep attachment to my father, came to visit almost on a monthly basis for a period of years. She also tried her best to get into Boston, to the MGH, in order to see Daddy on the night he died; but the morphine drip outpaced her. I was thankful for everything my sister and her daughters did to overcome the obstacles of distance.

Finally, I need to speak again of my gratitude to Julia Walker, not only for the love she gave my parents but also for the help she's given me in filling out pieces of the story that she remembers much more clearly than I do and for going through some of these pages with me to correct my errors. She was a blessing in my parents' lives, and now in mine. Thank you, Julia, for long years of friendship.

NOTES

CHAPTER 1

3   TEACHING ASSISTANT WHO HELPED MY FATHER WITH HIS
     WRITING: Michael Meyer, a poet and religious scholar,
     had known my father for a number of years, so there was
     a bond of trust that he could build on in the early stages
     of my father's illness.

3ff. MY FATHER'S SELF-DIAGNOSIS AND RELUCTANCE TO SHARE
      THIS INFORMATION WITH MY MOTHER: Naturally, he did
      discuss this with my mother in due time. I took it as a
      matter of trust not to pressure him.

CHAPTER 2

15   "RELIGION AND INSANITY": My father's senior honors the-
     sis was written in 1927 under the direction of Dr. Mor-
     ton Prince, a noted specialist in abnormal psychology
     who taught at Harvard College from 1926 to 1928.

17   EUGENE O'NEILL'S TREMOR MISDIAGNOSED AS PARKIN-
     SON'S DISEASE: My father believed the tremor was
     primarily the consequence of a form of neurological
     degeneration which, on the basis of O'Neill's family
     history, appeared to be hereditary. According to the au-
     topsy and neuropathological assessment of O'Neill car-
     ried out, at Carlotta's request, on November 28, 1953,
     there was no evidence of Parkinson's disease. "From
     time to time," the neuropathologist noted, "various
     drugs regularly used for the control of Parkinsonism had
     been tried, but these invariably made him worse."

18   DEATH OF EUGENE O'NEILL: According to a memo that
     my father wrote on November 30, 1953, "Eugene died
     on Friday, November 27 at 4:39 p.m. He died in his own
     bed in his apartment at the Hotel Shelton....I had pre-

dicted in the morning that he would go with the sunset and so he did." The cause of his death, my father wrote, was bronchial pneumonia. O'Neill's burial was on December 1, 1953, at Forest Hills Cemetery in Boston.

19 ALFRED NORTH WHITEHEAD: My father said he took Professor Whitehead's philosophy course in 1924. He also said he sometimes visited Whitehead at his home along with other students on a Sunday afternoon. I have no way to confirm this.

CHAPTER 3

34 MY FATHER STILL READING MEDICAL JOURNALS: In late June 1999, I noticed that my father had underlined the title and the first few lines of an article on Alzheimer's disease that he had found in *The British Journal of Neurology*. He had been in the nursing home nearly three years at the time.

42 "REPAIR REPETITIONS": My father's memo is condensed to bypass words that I could not decipher or where their meaning was obscure. I've followed the same practice elsewhere in the book in cases where I couldn't read some portions of his writing or where he meandered into pleasant but irrelevant digressions.

CHAPTER 4

65, 66 "ONEIRIC STATE," "EMERGENT PROPERTIES," SPONTANEOUS ELECTRICAL EVENTS: The physician who explained this to me also used the term "spontaneous firing of the circuits" in reference to the activation of a memory or a small piece of a memory. For a more extensive explanation of what may appear to us to be emerging memories, see Daniel Schacter, cited in note for Chapter 12, p. 235.

CHAPTER 5

75 APPARENT DERELICTION OF MEDICAL DIRECTOR AT NURSING HOME: There was more than one medical director

during the years my father stayed there. My reference
here is to the physician who filled this role at the time
my father underwent this crisis.

77 MY FATHER'S USE OF AN ELECTROENCEPHALOGRAM TO
IDENTIFY LOCATION OF A CYST ON THE RIGHT SIDE OF A
WOMAN'S BRAIN: The E.E.G. (which is no longer used for
this diagnostic purpose) did not show the image of a cyst
or tumor. What it showed were fluctuating brain waves,
indicating variations in electrical activity in different
sections of the brain. By examination of the E.E.G. a
doctor could surmise the probable location and approx-
imate dimensions of a cyst or other lesion.

87ff. DR. MERRILL MOORE'S BRILLIANCE, ECCENTRICITY, AND
ASSOCIATIONS IN THE WORLD OF THEATER: Among his
most successful cases was that of Joshua Logan, a prominent theatrical director in New York, whom Dr. Moore
treated for severe depression. In his memoirs, Logan
wrote that, when he had a consultation, "Merrill would
lope in and autograph one of his books...to me....I
avoided reading them, but I couldn't avoid his reciting
them to me, which he did constantly while walking down
halls or going up in elevators. He told me he composed
his sonnets while crossing streets or climbing stairs or
while he was starting his car." See Joshua Logan, *Josh*
(New York: Delacorte Press, 1976).

89–91 MY FATHER'S EXAMINATION OF CARLOTTA AND MEETING
WITH O'NEILL: According to my father's notes and a
dictation tape he made, he was called into the case by
the clinical director of McLean, who believed there
was a "concerted plan" to terminate Carlotta's marriage, "and immobilize her, so to speak [my father's
words] under the guise of involuntary hospitalization."
The director also told him that Carlotta had been
brought to McLean from Salem Hospital, close to the
town of Marblehead, where the couple had been living. She had been admitted to the hospital in February 1951, because of confusion attributed to bromide
poisoning, which was at first mistaken for hysteria.
O'Neill, my father said, was also at the hospital during
this period, because he had a broken leg from having fallen outside of his home in Marblehead after a
stormy quarrel with Carlotta. While O'Neill was still

in Salem Hospital, Dr. Moore induced him to sign the petition alleging that Carlotta was insane. My father's first meeting with O'Neill was, he said, in early May "at the Doctors' Hospital in New York," where O'Neill was being treated for pneumonia.

CHAPTER 6

104   MY FATHER INJURING HIMSELF AT NURSING HOME: "At 6:20 a.m. Harry fell. He was found lying on floor next to his bed," according to a nurse's note. "He sustained an abrasion above his left eyebrow."

106, 107   MY MOTHER AND THE RED SOX: In 1918, the previous time the Red Sox won the World Series, my mother was fourteen. When they won again in 2004, my mother kept on telling Julia, "Yes! They won! I saw it!" She asked Julia to put up pictures of her favorite players on the bedroom wall.

107   GIRLS' LATIN SCHOOL: Technically, according to official records, the school was never closed but was transformed in 1971 into a new and very different coeducational institution and given a new name.

CHAPTER 7

120   EUGENE O'NEILL'S LAST WILL AND TESTAMENT: The copy I found in my father's desk was dated June 28, 1948. According to a letter from my father to Robert Meserve, a Boston attorney retained by Carlotta, the 1948 will was superseded by a new will, dated March 5, 1951, which O'Neill signed at Merrill Moore's urging while Carlotta was in McLean and which was subsequently revoked and replaced by a third and, I believe, final will later the same year.

120–122   BLEMIE'S WILL: The Last Will and Testament of Silverdene Emblem O'Neill, which I first read in a typed version, was dated "Tao House, December 17, 1940." Six years after O'Neill's death, Carlotta sent my father a privately printed copy of the will, which she inscribed to me "from O'Neill and Blemie and Carlotta."

122ff.   QUOTATIONS BY MY FATHER FROM EUGENE O'NEILL, AL-
TERCATIONS BETWEEN O'NEILL AND CARLOTTA, O'NEILL'S
EXPRESSIONS OF REMORSE IN REFERENCE TO HIS DAUGH-
TER: The primary sources, here and elsewhere in this
book, are my father's handwritten notes and typed
transcripts of more extensive notes he made while he
was talking with O'Neill or shortly afterward, as well
as his later observations, reflections, and summations,
which he would dictate periodically. His initial and
subsequent conversations with Oona at her home in
Switzerland are documented in his notes and in their
correspondence.

124   PATRICIA NEAL AUDITIONED FOR ONE OF O'NEILL'S PLAYS:
The play was *A Moon for the Misbegotten,* which toured
several cities in 1947 but was not produced on Broadway
in the playwright's lifetime. Ms. Neal spoke about her
meetings with O'Neill and their friendship with each
other in her autobiographical book *As I Am* (New York:
Simon and Schuster, 1988).

125   PATRICIA NEAL'S CAREER AND CEREBRAL IMPAIRMENT:
The actress, who received an Academy Award for her
role in *Hud* in 1964, suffered a brain hemorrhage in 1965
but successfully resumed her career in 1968, according
to her obituary in *The New York Times,* August 9, 2010.

126   CARLOTTA VETOED MY FATHER'S SUGGESTION THAT HE
AND O'NEILL MIGHT GO TO SEE A GAME AT FENWAY PARK:
According to my father's notes, she followed up on this
by telling the staff at the hotel that O'Neill "was not to
leave the building without her express instructions."

129   THE BETTER PART OF TWO AND A HALF YEARS: My father's
treatment of O'Neill began in mid-May 1951 and continued until the playwright's death on November 27, 1953.

CHAPTER 8

148   DIFFICULTIES SILVIA AND JULIA FACED IN TRYING TO MAKE
CONTACT WITH MY FATHER'S DOCTOR: "We never know,"
Julia said, "if the answers that we finally get from someone in the office are based on the information we provided. I mean, we don't know if the doctor herself ever
got that information. Sometimes they tell us, 'The doctor

hasn't had a chance to look at the lab results yet,' or some other answer we were waiting for, 'but we'll be in touch tomorrow.' Then, the next day, they might say, 'He does have an infection, so we called in a prescription. You can go and pick it up.' But we still don't know if the doctor is aware of this. We have to push too hard...."

154   INSUFFICIENT NUMBER OF GERIATRICIANS: "Medical schools and residencies require little to no geriatric training, and many students are reluctant to get into the field because it is among the lowest paid in medicine....In 2005, there was one geriatrician for every 5,000 people over 65, according to the American Geriatrics Society; by 2030 that ratio is expected to increase to one for every 8,000 patients" (*The New York Times,* August 24, 2009). By way of contrast, there was one pediatrician for every 1,400 children in 2010 (op/ed by Dr. Dennis Rosen, *The New York Times,* July 22, 2010). The American Geriatrics Society (www.american geriatrics.org) is a primary source of updated news and academic research relevant to healthcare for the elderly. Its monthly publication, *Journal of the American Geriatric Society,* is written for specialists and scholars in the field, but I've found it helpful in understanding challenges confronting eldercare physicians and strategies to increase their numbers.

CHAPTER 9

166   EFFORTS BY FBI TO DISCREDIT DR. MARTIN LUTHER KING: See, for example, David Garrow, "The F.B.I. and Martin Luther King," *The Atlantic,* July 2002, and William Safire in *The New York Times,* November 20, 1975.

167   MY FATHER'S CAUTIONARY STATEMENT TO THE PROSECUTION IN THE TRIAL OF PATRICIA HEARST: "I have never made a commitment in advance of my own intensive study of the case and any opinion I may come up with is reached without regard to the side which may have retained me. It seems to me that the oath one takes to tell the truth and the whole truth and nothing but the truth is retrospective and encompasses the clinical study of

the subject from its very inception" (Letter from my father to U.S. Attorney James Browning and his colleague David Bancroft, October 14, 1975).

167 MY FATHER'S RECORDS OF HIS CONVERSATIONS WITH PATRICIA HEARST: The notes he made during, and just after, each conversation are written in very small and densely crowded script. A sixty-three-page typed version of these notes includes his commentary and reflections.

167 MY FATHER'S TESTIMONY: The official transcript of the proceedings in *United States v. Patricia Campbell Hearst* is reproduced in *The Trial of Patricia Hearst* (San Francisco: Great Fidelity Press, 1976).

168 PATRICIA'S ALLEGED MISTREATMENT AS A CHILD: "Now, I don't say that this is what happened, I wasn't there," my father testified. "This is her own image of what the first years of her life were...." He added that "she had a mixed picture of her childhood. She did have pets, a great deal of indulgence, and a great deal of freedom in many respects."

169 THE ABSENCE OF THE CLOSET IN PATRICIA'S DRAWING: The defense had emphasized the traumatic effect of a period of several weeks in which she said she had been held in a small closet by her captors. In the drawing, my father testified, she indicated where the kitchen and bathroom were, and the bedroom-living room, and she drew "two lines, diagonal lines..., to indicate where the two front windows were." She said the room had a large closet, which had two doors that opened and where a Murphy bed was kept. "And so she drew the two doors where the closet was, where the bed was kept, and she told me later that they kept much of the armament that they had there." He said she did not indicate any smaller closet in the drawing. (*The Trial of Patricia Hearst,* cited above. See also *San Francisco Chronicle,* March 16, 1976.) In my father's notes from his interview with Patricia on January 22, 1976, one of five interviews that totaled about sixteen hours, I found what is apparently an exact copy of Patricia's drawing. It's a very simple sketch. She drew large circles to indicate the rooms and parallel lines to represent the windows and the large closet in which the armaments were kept.

171   PATRICIA WONDERED IF HER LAWYER, F. LEE BAILEY, HAD BEEN DRINKING: In her book *Patty Hearst: Her Own Story,* written with Alvin Moscow (New York: Avon Books, 1988), Patricia said, "He rose from the defense table, grabbing an unruly stack of notes, and I could see that his hands were shaking...and his face was flushed. I wondered if he had been drinking at lunch....He spoke for less than forty-five minutes, but as I cringed in my seat, trying to follow his disjointed discourse, it seemed like a lifetime." See also *The Boston Evening Globe,* August 3, 1978.

171   OBITUARIES EMPHASIZED MY FATHER'S ROLE IN HEARST TRIAL: On the other hand, *The New York Times Magazine* (December 28, 2008), in a year-end issue devoted to twenty-four people who had passed away that year, gave a brief but warm portrayal of the trust his patients placed in him, exemplified in his close relationship with Eugene O'Neill.

176, 177   VICTORIA CHAPLIN: The man with whom she "ran away" (my mother's words) and whom she subsequently married, is Jean-Baptiste Thiérrée. Together, they created a circus performance, originally known as Le Cirque Imaginaire and later as Le Cirque Invisible.

CHAPTER 10

193   MY FATHER'S MEETING WITH EUGEN BLEULER: Dr. Bleuler had retired as director of the Burghölzli sanatorium in 1927, two years before my father's visit, but continued to receive foreign visitors there. After their meeting, he took my father to a smaller sanatorium in the nearby town of Küsnacht where he kept his private patients. It was there that my father was permitted to sit in on consultations and accompany the doctors when they were examining their patients. Dr. Bleuler's home, according to my father's notes and my mother's memory, was in a town called Zollikon.

202   RESIDENT SETTING UP MORPHINE DRIP: This must have been very early in the morning. I made a note that "my mother passed at 8:12 a.m."

CHAPTER 11

211 OTHER PEOPLE WORKING IN ASSOCIATION WITH MY FA-
THER'S DOCTOR WERE MORE RESPONSIVE TO HIS NEEDS
AND TO MESSAGES FROM SILVIA AND JULIA: After my father
returned from the hospital, a visiting nurse came to see
him once a week and a phlebotomist came twice a month
to take samples of his blood, apparently by arrangement
with his doctor's office. At this point, according to Julia,
she and Silvia did receive some belated guidance from
his doctor in helping him recover from the ulcer.

212 MY FATHER'S LETTER OF CRITIQUE OF DR. MEYER'S CLINIC:
He wrote this in August 1941 to Dr. John Whitehorn,
who replaced Dr. Meyer as director of the Phipps Clinic
on September 1, 1941.

216 MY FATHER RECOMMENDED A PSYCHOANALYST IN BOS-
TON WHO HAD BEEN DIRECTOR OF FREUD'S OUTPATIENT
DEPARTMENT: The man in question was Dr. Eduard
Hitschmann, who directed the Ambulatorium, which
was Freud's free or low-cost psychoanalytic clinic, from
1922 until he fled the Nazis in 1938, moving first to London, then to Boston in 1940.

217 THIRTEEN WOMEN STRANGLED IN OR CLOSE TO BOSTON: It
was originally believed that there were eleven victims,
but DeSalvo later confessed to two additional murders.
In his book *The Boston Strangler* (New York: New American Library, 1966), journalist Gerold Frank lists the
names and ages of all thirteen women. Five of them were
between nineteen and twenty-three; the other eight were
fifty-five or older.

217 DESCRIPTION IN PRESS ACCOUNT OF VICTIMS' BODIES: See
retrospective article by Loretta McLaughlin in *The Boston Globe,* June 7, 1992.

218 MY FATHER WAS ASKED BY THE COURT TO INTERVIEW DE-
SALVO: In a letter of April 6, 1965, my father told the
Massachusetts Commissioner of Mental Health that, "in
accordance with an order of the Honorable Arthur E.
Whittemore, Justice of the Supreme Judicial Court," the
examination of the mental condition of Albert H. De-
Salvo had been completed and that a transcript of the
interviews would shortly be available.

221 MY FATHER'S OPINION WAS OVERRULED BY OTHERS IN THE MENTAL HEALTH DEPARTMENT: Unlike those who disagreed with him, he was not asked to testify.

221 THE COMPETENCY DECISION: The hearing took place in June 1966, and the court's ruling was handed down in early July. The question of competency came up again in a pretrial hearing on January 10, 1967. The trial itself began the following day. (*The Boston Globe,* July 12, 2013.)

221 MY FATHER VIEWED THE COMPETENCY DECISION AS ILLOGICAL AND SELF-CONTRADICTORY: According to F. Lee Bailey, who was DeSalvo's lawyer (and would later represent Patricia Hearst), the decision of the court was, in part, the consequence of negotiations he had carried out with the prosecution. Bailey later explained the rather labyrinthine strategy that led him to agree to this apparent compromise. See *The Defense Never Rests,* by F. Lee Bailey with Harvey Aronson (New York: Stein and Day, 1971). See also *Time* magazine, January 27, 1969.

222, 223 DESALVO'S LETTER TO MY FATHER: DeSalvo's statement that "all of what has happen[ed] could have been avoided" if he had been under my father's direct supervision, while he was in detention, is difficult to understand, because the strangulations had, of course, taken place before the time when he was under observation. This is only one of several aspects of the letter that remain perplexing; but DeSalvo's professed sense of affection for my father seems to be authentic.

225 DESALVO'S GUILT: In 2013, a process known as DNA "familial searching" indicated a match between DeSalvo's DNA and a sample of DNA found on the body of a nineteen-year-old woman who was believed to be his final victim. (*The Boston Globe,* July 12, 2013.)

CHAPTER 12

235 THE RECONSTRUCTION OF MEMORIES: According to Schacter, "we tend to think of memories as snapshots from family albums that, if stored properly, could be retrieved in precisely the same condition in which they were put away. But we now know that we do not record

our experiences the way a camera records them. Our memories work differently. We extract key elements from our experiences and store them. We then recreate or restructure our experiences rather than retrieve copies of them. Sometimes, in the process of reconstructing we add on feelings, beliefs, or even knowledge we obtained after the experience. In other words, we bias our memories of the past by attributing to them emotions or knowledge we acquired after the event." See *The Seven Sins of Memory: How the Mind Forgets and Remembers,* by Daniel L. Schacter (New York: Houghton Mifflin Harcourt, 2001) and "The Cognitive Neuroscience of Constructive Memory," by Daniel Schacter and Donna Rose Addis, in *Philosophical Transactions of the Royal Society: Biological Sciences,* May 2007.

236 VICTORIA'S DAUGHTER, AURÉLIA, RECALLED HER DINNERS WITH HER MOTHER AND MY PARENTS: In one of my father's memos to himself, dated June 21, 1990, he said that he had met Victoria that evening, "following her appearance at the American Repertory Theater in Le Cirque Imaginaire. Met her husband, daughter, and son. Long conversation about Oona...." Aurélia has since become a star in her own right, touring internationally in an extraordinary one-woman performance, a continually evolving work of visual theater based on optical illusions, presented with an utterly original aesthetic sensibility, developed by Aurélia and Victoria. See also note for Chapter Nine, p. 176, "VICTORIA CHAPLIN."

EPILOGUE: 2015

247 HARVARD UNDERGRADUATES RANKED NUMERICALLY ON BASIS OF THEIR GRADES: According to the Harvard University Archives, this practice began in the early nineteenth century and ended at some point in the 1960s.

248, 249 FIRST MARSHAL: I can no longer remember exactly what it was that the first marshal did at the time of our commencement. At present, according to the secretary of Harvard's Phi Beta Kappa chapter, the first marshals lead the procession at literary exercises held a few days prior to commencement.

256   MY BOOK ABOUT ADULT NONREADERS AND THEIR CHIL-
DREN: *Illiterate America* (New York: Doubleday, 1985).

258   A CHILD BEATEN WITH A BAMBOO WHIP: I described this
child and other children in my class in *Death at an Early
Age* (Boston: Houghton Mifflin, 1967).

259   MY INDECISION ABOUT MOVING INTO ACADEMIC LIFE:
Looking back, I wonder why I felt convinced that I
would lose something I valued if I crossed the line between two social settings. Hundreds of activists who
made this move continued to be loyal to the interests
of low-income children and their parents, and perhaps
were more effective advocates because their academic
roles may have accorded them more credibility. I think,
in the long run, it was the question of physical and emotional vantage point that held me back. I continued to
live in the same urban neighborhood for approximately
eighteen years.

269   MY FATHER'S PRIMARY PHYSICIAN DECLARED HIM INCA-
PABLE OF MANAGING HIS AFFAIRS: This was in February
1996. Remarkably, as late as April 25, my father wrote
to me that he was hoping to take my mother back to
Europe for a final time. Six weeks later, he was in the
nursing home.

INDEX

About the Author

JONATHAN KOZOL received the National Book Award in Science, Philosophy, and Religion for *Death at an Early Age*, the Robert F. Kennedy Book Award for *Rachel and Her Children*, and countless other honors for *Savage Inequalities*, *Amazing Grace*, and his most recent writings about poverty and childhood. For more information, visit www.jonathankozol.com.

Also by Jonathan Kozol

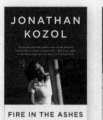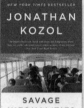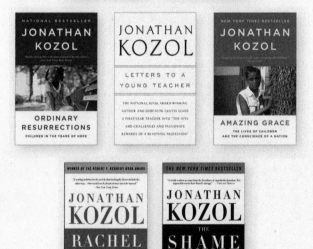

B \ D \ W \ Y

Available wherever books are sold